Hot Water for Tea

Hot Water for Tea

An inspired collection of tea remedies and aromatic elixirs
For your mind and body, beauty and soul

NICOLA SALTER

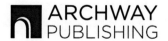

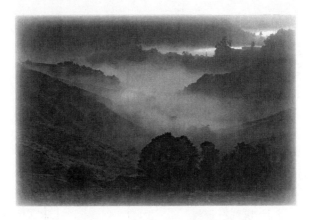

Copyright © 2013 Nicola J Salter.

Archway Publishing books may be ordered through booksellers or by contacting:

Archway Publishing
1663 Liberty Drive
Bloomington, IN 47403
www.archwaypublishing.com
1-(888)-242-5904

Because of the dynamic nature of the Internet, any web addresses or links contained in this book may have changed since publication and may no longer be valid. The views expressed in this work are solely those of the author and do not necessarily reflect the views of the publisher, and the publisher hereby disclaims any responsibility for them.

Disclaimer: It is as the reader's discretion how they follow the guidelines in this book. Neither the author nor the publisher can be held responsible for any adverse reactions to the recipes, recommendations and instructions contained herein. As always please consult your primary health care provider in cases of serious or long-term health issues and during pregnancy, before following the recipes contained in this book, which are not intended to diagnose, treat, cure, or prevent any disease.

Cover Photo © National Geographic/Eliza R. Skidmore

ISBN: 978-1-4808-0248-3 (e)
ISBN: 978-1-4808-0247-6 (sc)
ISBN: 978-1-4808-0249-0 (hc)

Library of Congress Control Number: 2013918127

Printed in the United States of America

Archway Publishing rev. date: 10/18/2013

For Olivia
My Niece

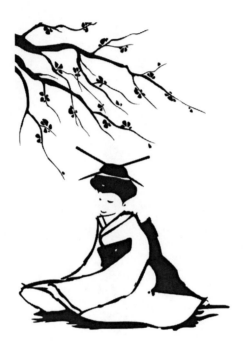

Willow branches graze the grass,
As I sit in the shade drinking tea.
A note from a flute blows clearly,
Mingling with the sound of rain.
 I could sit here alone forever,
 And still I'd never feel lonely.

Anonymous poem inscribed on an
ancient Yi Hsing teapot

With love and grateful thanks

First of all to the many dear friends and colleagues who gave so much of their time to help me with this book, I thank you.

Special thanks go to my mum, for her love, innate wisdom and who taught me to understand the power of food as medicine, and to:

Pete, for being a willing tester of my tea cocktails, for his research and layout of the photographs and his time and dedication spent on the front cover for this book, and most of all for his love and for sharing his life with me.

Julia, for her love, inspiration and encouragement to follow my dreams.

Olivia, for her love and delicious cupcake recipe and for bringing so much joy into my world.

Joe Whitehead, for her infinite knowledge of history and antiques.

Susan and Bob, Sarah and Nancy, for their dear friendship and support.

Jacqueline Kidd, gifted naturopath, for her generosity, skill and ability to help so many regain their health and their lives.

Kathy Long, a dear friend and gifted acupuncturist, who generously assisted with testing formulations, and also to her daughter, Kara, for her green tea ice cream recipe.

And dear friend Anna Marie de la Fuente, for her editing expertise and drive to help me get the book finished on time, and to Marie Zapien for her time and editing input.

A sincere thanks to all those who made a beautiful and lasting impact on my life:

Terry Moule, D.O., N.D., Alan Protheroe, Terry Lowe and especially, my Dad.

Table of Contents

Foreword

You hold in your hands a serendipitous invitation to embrace your well-being, and nurture your soul. It is an invitation to enjoy a time-honored tradition that dates back over four thousand years, still holding relevance today. In her debut literary work, Nicola Salter delights us with the perfect balance of charming anecdotes, clinical applications, and practical experience. *Hot Water for Tea* beckons us to cultivate tranquility, to take a pause in the daily scheme and realize a connection with ourselves and those around us.

As a natural health consultant and educator for over fourteen years, I have had the good fortune to have Nicola Salter as an esteemed colleague. I have personally witnessed remarkable transformations in her clients' awareness and well-being. Her knowledge and dedication in assisting others reach their higher self is evident throughout the pages of *Hot Water for Tea*. From the tea leaf's humble beginnings to its use in noble ceremonies across the globe, Nicola takes us on a mindful journey, awakening our senses and our palates. She graciously enlightens us with the techniques for creating the perfect cup of tea, in taste, fragrance and color for every occasion. Discover how to balance the amount of caffeine present in each cup of tea you savor, which teas and essential oils will deliver sought-after health benefits, and which ones to avoid. Her research is detailed and relevant, appealing to both health professionals and non-professionals alike.

Going beyond the "humble tea leaf", Nicola includes the fruits of her many years as a noted and acclaimed clinical aromatherapist with health-promoting elixirs for mind and body. Nicola shares the multi-faceted healing capabilities of essential oils, that when combined with tea, take our simple cup of "cha" to a whole new level.

Hot Water for Tea is an invitation I welcome you to accept for harmony, for grace and for life.

Jacqueline Kidd Ph.D.,N.P.
Director, Calabasas Center for Natural Health
Co-founder, Options for Life Foundation

About the Author

Nicola Salter was born in London, the daughter of parents whose fondness for using natural foods as a preventative health measure inspired her to train for a career in wellness: focusing on clinical aromatherapy, energy medicine and Japanese *Reiki*. She served for a number of years outside the complementary health field, working for the BBC and large corporations, where she specialized in marketing, public relations and the media.

Nicola and her sister Julia were raised in a naturopathic household, where natural remedies ruled whenever medicinal treatment was required. Nicola commends her parents for instilling in her a passion for natural health and learning at an early age how to use natural ingredients for skin and health care. Today, her own home transmits the same feel of holistic wellness. She also conveys this feeling at her private practices in Calabasas and Woodland Hills, California where for the past 17 years she has built an extensive client base as an intuitive counselor, energy-medicine practitioner, and coach, working alongside both Eastern and Western health practices supporting clients to better manage life's challenges, encouraging them with inspirational tools to uncover and discover their true essence. The formulations you find in this book have been created and used by Nicola for her clients.

In addition to her clinical practice, Nicola also teaches the art of Japanese *Reiki*, clinical aromatherapy, the spirit of aromatherapy and energy healing methods. She has promoted her own effective home remedies on both television and radio; created an award-winning aromatherapy skincare line, and her product-line, "Clear," has achieved laudatory reviews from therapists in traditional and alternative medicine.

Of all those who have shone brightly for Nicola, naturopaths Terry Moule, D.O., N.D. and Roderick Lane, N.D. are two stars for whom Nicola is forever grateful, for their patience, their encouragement and their support.

Nicola Salter can be reached at: www.nicolasalter.com

Introduction to a World of Fragrance

Ever since I was a child, scents, taste and ceremony have always held a fascination for me.

Fragrances evoke memories and feelings: whether they be that of fresh chocolate; carnations and burning candles at a church wedding; freshly cut grass; rosemary and lavender bushes; the heat on the airport tarmac as you step out to a new adventure; porridge in Scotland; the Edinburgh Railway Station; an old book; new clothes. I am sure you can add to the list.

A few years after I moved to Los Angeles, the aroma of orange blossom was so overwhelming that I thought no other fragrance would ever replace it. But one day, while out shopping, it was the delightful and surprisingly aromatic cloud of fruits, herbs and spices that lured me into a tea store. Just as the smell of bread entices your taste buds, it was the same for me with tea.

I had experienced the heady bazaars of Egypt with their spices and mint teas; the floral sweet smells of Beirut; the grassy clean aroma of *mate* tea in Bolivia, and the fantastic fragrances of essential oils bursting out of their mysterious dark bottles, but on this particular day, the scent of this aromatic cloud had a purpose and was drawing me to it.

The tea store was a well-known retail chain of U.K. tea suppliers, and that day was truly a catalyst for me. It was a day to wake up and discover a treasure trove of delicious tea elixirs.

Since I'm British, one might assume I am a natural tea drinker, but this isn't the case. I had been drinking and recommending herbal teas for years with my clients but until that moment, my taste buds had not experienced an *oolong*, a really good quality green or white tea, or even a *pu'erh* tea. At that time I had never even heard of yellow tea.

The store manager appeared fascinated by my excitement. My senses began to rapidly match the scents and characteristics of essential oils with the selection of teas she presented to me. Finally, my brain calmed down and we talked about holding an event for shoppers to discover the health benefits of essential oils and teas.

In truth, the event we held at the store was the beginning of this book.

Of course, the subject of tea has turned out to be extremely comprehensive. Combined with aromatherapy, these are two weighty subjects. There is definitely so much more I could have included. However, my intention is to give simple hands-on information and not to overwhelm you, the reader.

What began as a light exploration and creation of remedies has culminated in a profoundly soulful journey for me. You see, the art of tea, whichever way you drink it, or whichever country you come from, has one underlining thread for all of us. It is the cultivation of yourself as you come to understand and follow the ceremony of mindful attention for tea preparation; the focus, the way in which you take your tea, and where you drink it; the respect for others as you fill their cups with grace follow a timeless tradition. It all adds up to a delightful meditation, contemplation, a space for just being and not doing, and the chance for meaningful conversation with others.

Through the ceremony of tea, I realized the correlation with *Reiki* that I have taught for many years. *Reiki* is the Japanese art of energy renewal for expanding our consciousness and for self-healing as well healing others. Through the discipline of *Reiki*, I came to value and understand the place for ceremony and ritual in our busy world; to help us transform through the daily practice of movement, meditation, *Reiki,* and now also tea.

The art of aromatherapy continues the process of self-discovery. As you create the blends from this book, using oils extracted from plants, fruits, herbs and roots, you are working with nature to focus on how the essential oil makes you feel by its aroma, its character, and how it could soothe a headache or help you sleep. You become deeply quiet and reflective as you pour the oils into the bottle, mixing and defining, and redefining the blend to meet your requirements.

As a result, it is the very essence of the flowers or herbs you have chosen that will bring out your true essence, defining and redefining who *you* are.

Nature's medicine cabinet provides us with many tools for good, healthy and simple living. Combine these tools with meditation and ceremony and we have the opportunity to thrive no matter how busy we may be.

I invite you to join me in a cup of tea to nourish your body and soul.

Wishing you a very good life.

As always
Nicola

Using this Book for your Well-being

In writing this book, I decided that I would feel more comfortable writing about teas I had thoroughly researched and experienced for myself and with my clients.

A large percentage of tea research is done in a petri dish or on rats. As yet, human studies are not as abundant. You will see detailed research reports at the back of the book if you wish to follow up for your own reference.

Hot Water for Tea covers traditional teas, including black, green *matcha*, white, yellow, *oolong* and *pu'erh* along with a variety of herbal tisanes that can be combined with the traditional teas mentioned above. In addition, the use of certain essential oils combined with tea really brings home a truly health-giving aromatic drink and gives you the opportunity to become quite the tea artisan!

For herbal teas not included in this book, you will find many excellent books written on the healing benefits of herbs.

I hope this book introduces you effectively -and in an enjoyable way - to tea remedies and essential oil blends for specific health issues. I would recommend - in cases where your health issues are more complicated - to find a qualified herbalist, Chinese medicine practitioner or naturopath.

Nature's apothecary has given us fresh plants, fruits, flowers and roots from which we extract our potent essential oils, and the simple tea bush for our healing teas. Enjoy your journey of self-discovery as you explore the pleasures of tea and aromatherapy for your mind, body and spirit.

Hot Water for Tea

The Story of the Humble Tea Leaf

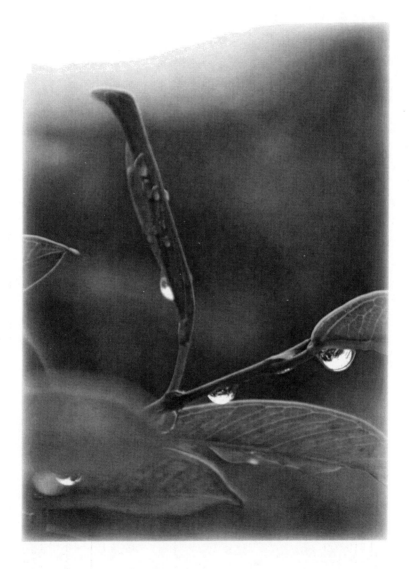

"Tea is a cup of Life."
Anonymous

The Story of the Humble Tea Leaf

Long ago, tea was only available to the nobility owing to its expense, and it became known as "the noble leaf." Noble it is, mighty it is and at the same time, humble.

Tea to this day remains a drink for all people, leaders and workers alike, bringing us together no matter what the situation as we enjoy our daily cup of *cha* to relax and warm our spirits. Tea has been quietly constant for thousands of years, bringing us its healing benefits and even changing the course of history.

Quite simply, from nature to your cup, the humble tea leaf gives so much and asks only that you simply enjoy it.

Long before coffee was discovered, legend has it that in 2737 B.C.E (before the common era, before Christ), while Chinese Emperor Shen-Nung was travelling with his army, he inadvertently created the first cup of tea.

The emperor always had his drinking water boiled, and on one particular day, the servant preparing it didn't see a dried leaf fall into the water from the nearby wild tea bush. The water turned brown and Shen-Nun, being quite the herbalist, decided to sample it and found the water to be refreshing and energizing. In that moment tea or *cha* was born, and today 2.5 million tons of tea is produced in over forty countries. The little tea leaf has come a very long way since its discovery.

Interestingly, the British still refer to tea as *cha*. Frequently you will hear folks saying, "Let's put the kettle on" or "Have a cup of *cha*," often when they need to work out a problem or want to put their feet up for a few minutes, hence the celebrated British tea break.

The word *cha* didn't come into recorded existence until 760 C.E. when a scholar named Lu Yu wrote the *Cha Jing*, meaning *The Classic of Tea*." Up until then, tea was actually called *tu* or *jia*, which later evolved into "tea" or "chai."

China is considered to have the earliest records of tea drinking, dating back to the first millennium B.C.E. and then to the Han Dynasty (206 B.C.E.– 20 C.E.) which used tea as medicine. This was followed by the Tan Dynasty (618-907 C.E.) where they drank tea for pleasure and during social events.

Tea was often used as "food" in a broth, or for ceremonies, with the exchange of tea gifts: either teacakes or bricks of tea. Chinese Daoists referred to tea as "the elixir of immortality" and eventually, tea became one of the seven essentials of daily life.

During 794-1195 C.E. Japanese monks had already recognized the importance of tea during their travels to China; returning with seeds for tea bushes and slowly cultivating tea for themselves and the nobility. However, it wasn't until 1191 C.E. that a Japanese monk, Eisai, who studied Zen Buddhism in China, brought tea seeds back to Japan to grow larger numbers of tea bushes and make *matcha* green tea more widely available to the Japanese people and consequently wrote the first book on tea, *Drinking Tea for Health*.

Tea spread to the Arab countries and Africa as a major export from China to the Silk Road on land and sea. Tea leaves often replaced coins for trading, making the humble tea leaf a major player in establishing trade connections between the East and West.

Tea Arrives in Europe

In 1606, Dutch and Portuguese traders introduced tea to Europe where it rapidly became a popular alternative to coffee among wealthy Dutch women. Barred from the all-male ale and coffee houses, the women began to drink tea together at home.

Tea became such a must-have that the John Company traders and the Dutch East India Trade Company had quite the monopoly on the tea market, with their fast-sailing clippers bringing as much fresh tea as possible back from China to Europe for the new fashionable tea houses and the nobility. It was expensive to buy and only available to the rich.

Tea spread to Britain in 1657, and in 1658 a London newspaper advertised a new drink from China, called *tcha,* or *tay* (pronounced tee) that was on sale for the first time in a London coffeehouse.

At first tea was poorly prepared by the coffee houses, and they would often brew the tea with too much water for far too long and store it in beer barrels!

It was Queen Catherine of Braganza, originally from Portugal, who put tea on the map for England when she married King

Charles II. She was an avid tea drinker and by 1662, tea had become so popular that it overtook alcohol in the popularity stakes. By 1717, Thomas Twining opened his first teashop in London for both men and women - quite scandalous in those days!

Due to the heavy taxes placed on tea, it was still an expensive commodity and only available to the rich and upper class. In the homes of the wealthy, the lady of the house would carry a key on a ribbon tied around her waist to open the tea chest where the valuable tea was stored. Nobody else had access to this chest. She was allowed the first two brews of the tea leaves in her tea bowl. The housekeeper then got to brew the tea leaves again for herself and the servants, and then finally, peddlers would come by to purchase the very used and worn-out tea leaves to sell at local markets.

By the eighteenth century, many British people wanted to drink tea but couldn't afford it and the illegal trade of smuggling tea into Britain quickly grew in popular support. Things began to get out of hand when to maximize profits, smugglers began to adulterate tea with leaves from other plants or tea leaves that had been previously brewed. Even worse, they sometimes combined it with sheep's dung.

Prime Minister William Pitt the Younger (1759-1806) brought smuggling to an end but by then, the bootleggers had made a historical and lasting impact on the distribution of tea, which became available to everyone in Britain, and not just the nobility.

Tea became so entrenched in British society that 1930s author Nancy Mitford coined the phrase "my cup of tea" to describe a positive friendship. "She is just my cup of tea" became a phrase known to convey the strength, goodness and positive aspects of a person. It wasn't until World War II in 1944 that the phrase became less positive, and if Britons disliked someone, they'd say "he's not my cup of tea"rather than the American phrase "he's a pain in the neck.".

Tea Arrives in America

The Dutch East India Company evolved into the British East India Company, which by now had the monopoly on tea. It was in the eighteenth century when the company's first shipments of tea arrived in New York and Boston.

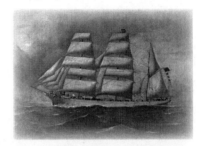

With increases in revenue and administration to get the tea to North America, and with debts accrued from the French and Indian wars, British Parliament enacted the Tea Act, placing heavier taxes on tea and other goods into the American colonies. This allowed Britain to ship tea from China straight to America and gave Britain the right to all sales on tea. Since the colonies were no longer under British rule, they boycotted the British goods and teas and refused to pay the taxes.

In 1773, seven ships from England arrived carrying tea, and the Bostonians were waiting, dressed as Native American Indians. They boarded one of the clippers, the Dartmouth, and threw its cargo of *lapsang souchong* tea into the sea. This marked the famous Boston Tea Party and heralded American independence. Once again, the tea leaf took its place in history along with a phrase coined by then British Prime Minister North (1770 - 1782) who referred to the whole affair as a "tempest in a teacup" which later became "a storm in a teacup."

Tea eventually reached India, when the British East India Company decided to look at new areas outside of China to cultivate and reliably produce tea. Trading of British goods with China for tea was beginning to wane, and being supplanted by the illegal trade of opium.

The British discovered that India provided an ideal temperate climate for growing tea, which would subsequently help India's economy, but prove devastating to China. In fact, coupled with the two Opium Wars between Britain and China during Queen Victoria's reign, the face of the tea trade dramatically changed and by 1860, 85 percent of tea came from India and Ceylon (now known as Sri Lanka), and only 12 percent from China.

The Invention of the Teacup

Tea was cheap at its source in China, and was drunk without much ceremony and quite casually from a cup without a handle, a tiny tea bowl made from ceramic material that held 30 ml of liquid.

The Japanese poured their tea with more ceremony but the Europeans, unlike their Asian counterparts, served their tea extremely hot so it would dissolve the sugar and consequently, the tea bowls became too hot to hold. This required the invention of the teacup handle. By the mid-eighteenth century, handle makers appeared in most cities.

In 1750, artisan Robert Adams began designing teacups with handles. The cups were taller and wider at the rim and also came with saucers. Adams made the cups from porcelain, which was strong but also delicate. He then went on to create sugar holders, teapots, and milk jugs to match.

In the late 1830s, tea reached new heights in Europe with wealthy ladies of the time taking afternoon tea with their delicate fine China tea services.

It is widely believed that Lady Bedford, who served as a Lady of the Bedchamber to her close friend Queen Victoria, introduced the afternoon tea ritual. She is said to have added delicate cakes and sandwiches to the already accepted tradition of afternoon tea, making it a light repast before dinner.

What is evident is that in the Western world, afternoon tea had begun to make its mark as an opportunity for showing the best of one's manners and a time for sharing with friends.

Present Day – The Ironic Turnaround

In what could only be described as a rather ironic turn of events in the history of our humble tea leaf, a new tea plantation has sprung up in England in recent years, and it appears that today the British are supplying the Chinese with tea.

The Tregothnan estate in Cornwall has an ideal micro-climate to grow the *Camellia sinensis* teabush owing to the air and humidity, which closely resemble the foothills of the Himalayas. The estate harvests 11.4 tons of tea leaves annually and now exports the tea to China where it has been widely accepted for its exquisite taste.

The humble tea leaf continues to meander along a journey of twists and turns, making its mark on history but in essence, untouched and unchanged. Its simplicity and symbolism of hospitality and graceful ceremony remain as constant today as when it was first discovered.

The Worldwide Ceremony of Tea
for
Harmony, Purity, Tranquility and Respect

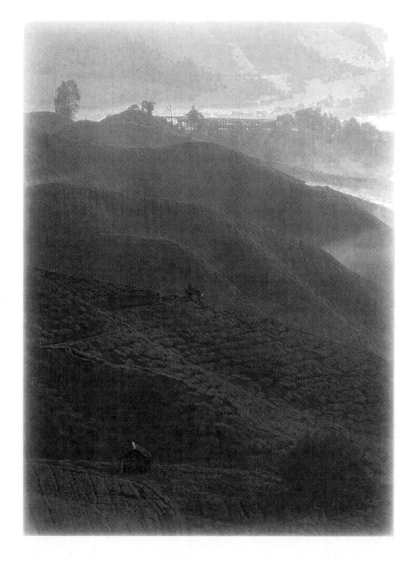

"Every encounter is once in a lifetime."
-Takeno Joo, 15ᵗʰc Tea Master

The Ceremony of Tea in a Busy World

Every time you make a cup of tea, you are repeating an ancient ritual of tranquility, harmony and hospitality. Whichever style of tea ceremony you choose will give you the chance to be still for a few moments, to listen to your inner thoughts and inspirations, and ultimately be rewarded with an uplifting blend of grassy or spicy notes.

Whether you are sipping tea from a mug in your kitchen, or from a porcelain tea cup with tiny sweet morsels in a fine establishment; or even farther afield in a Japanese tea house, a wedding in China; or sipping spicy chai in India or hot butter tea in Tibet, tea is perceived worldwide as a vital core of hospitality and friendship.

Cha dao - The Way of Tea in China

> *"Better to go three days without food than one day without tea."*
> *Old Chinese adage.*

Drinking tea in China is all about enjoying and discussing the flavor and fragrance of the chosen tea, and how it compares to another. The Chinese gather over tea to share thoughts and ideas as they drink together.

The Chinese tea ceremony is conducted to express gratitude, ask forgiveness, or instill goodwill among guests at family reunions or wedding celebrations.

Their tea ceremony is less formal than that of the Japanese, and the ritual of making and pouring the tea may be performed differently by each person serving the tea. Chinese tea bowls are much smaller than the Japanese ones, allowing only two small swallows of tea. However, the cups are larger in Shanghai and Beijing.

Both Chinese and Japanese tea ceremonies have their roots in Zen Buddhism. But while a Japanese tea ceremony gives guests the opportunity to sit in quiet reflection as the tea is prepared, the Chinese ceremony celebrates a coming together of people or an event, and the tea server will often relate positive and funny anecdotes to entertain the guests. During the Chinese ceremony, dried fruits are served with the tea while sweet candy snacks are served during the Japanese ritual.

In Chinese, *Gung Fu Cha* means "Tea with Great Skill" and those preparing and serving the tea are required to do so with the highest precision and consistency. Connoisseurs of fine tea are known as *cha-ren,* meaning "tea people," and they are very specific about the type of water used for the tea, the occasion, the time, the apparatus, and even their guests.

The *Kungfu* (meaning sophisticated and adept skills) tea ceremony is performed with a tiny teapot and cups the size of half tennis balls. The small tea service (*Yixing* teaware) enables tea to be served fresh and finished immediately. The cups are all placed together, and the tea is poured quickly to ensure the taste remains the same for each serving, and from a low height over each cup to prevent froth. It is customary to note the tea's color, taste and fragrance while drinking it.

Most of the teas consumed in China are grown in the mountains of Taiwan at 4,000 feet, making the teas, such as *oolong*, particularly refined, with excellent health benefits.

The following is an excerpt from an interview with Popchong Sunim at the Songgwang Sa monastery in Korea that perhaps best describes the art of tea in China. The full interview was posted on June 22, 2010 by *Buddhism Now*.

"… Do not gulp the tea but sip it slowly, allowing its fragrance to fill one's mouth. There is no need to have any special attitude while drinking, except one of thankfulness. The nature of the tea itself is that of no-mind. It does not discriminate and make differences. It is just as it is …"

"…Tea is drunk either to quench the thirst, savour the taste or simply to spend a quiet hour appreciating the pottery and the general atmosphere that accompanies tea drinking …"

The Ceremony of Tea in Japan

"The pleasure of the tea relies on the indescribable charm of a host conveying his or her deepest feeling to the guests by selecting the tea utensils and tableware, assorting and arranging things according to their due, the season and the theme…". - Sen Shoshitsu XV, Grand Master of the *Urasenke* Tradition of Tea.

In was in the fifteenth century when the Japanese introduced the practice of preparing green tea powder, *matcha,* as an art of performance and spiritual practice, called the "tea ceremony." Influenced by Zen Buddhism, the ceremony is, in essence, a form of meditation. Each part of the ceremony is done with great mindfulness and focus, paying careful attention to every movement and action: from whisking the tea, to pouring and then drinking it.

A historical figure in the creation of the tea ceremony was Sen No Rikyu who followed his master's belief system that each meeting should be treasured for it can never be reproduced. The tea ceremony called *chanoyu,* which translates into "hot water for tea," brings the qualities of respect, harmony, purity and tranquility into your life through the refined and ritualized making of *matcha.*

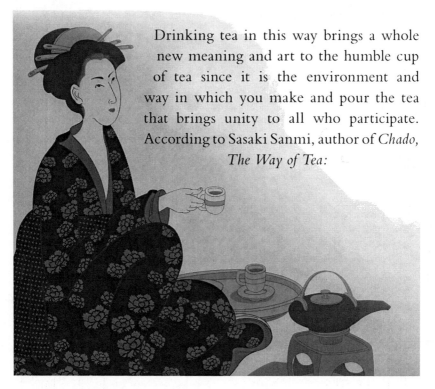

Drinking tea in this way brings a whole new meaning and art to the humble cup of tea since it is the environment and way in which you make and pour the tea that brings unity to all who participate. According to Sasaki Sanmi, author of *Chado, The Way of Tea:*

"The tea gathering must emphasize 'one time, one meeting' and must generate between the host and guest spiritual communication. This is so highly valued that a tea gathering, even with a gorgeous set of utensils and skillfully performed procedures, will not be highly rated unless there is spiritual unity."

The tea ceremony takes place in the *chashitsu* (tearoom) which is minimally decorated with calligraphy, poems, a single flower or grass stem to allow the guests to feel the beauty of the space and of nature while bonding over tea and *kaiseki* (sweet delicacies). Every element contributes to the enjoyment of the tea.

There are rules to the tea ceremony where every moment matters and is savored as it represents how we can give full attention to life in the moment. There are different types of tea ceremonies for each season.

Green Tea's Spiritual Debut

Japanese Zen Buddhist monk Eisai can be credited for bringing green tea to Japan, and for making the tea leaf a key part of the Japanese tea ceremony.

When Eisai returned from China circa 1191 C.E. after studying to become a Zen teacher, he brought back with him a large number of tea bush seeds and Zen scriptures. Much to the chagrin of the noblemen and priests who until then had exclusive use of the rare tea plant for medicinal uses, he grew and nurtured the bushes to make green tea more widely available to the population. He demonstrated how to make *matcha* by grinding the green tea leaves to a fine powder and mixing it with hot water. He was also accredited with cultivating and using tea for religious purposes other than just for medicine.

In Eisai's book *Tea Drinking for Health* (*Kissa yojoki*), he explained his belief that good health lies in the health of the five organs; the heart, liver, lungs, spleen and kidney. Drinking *matcha* could strengthen the heart and since the heart is the most superior of the organs, this would also improve the other organs.

Invitation to a Japanese Tea Ceremony

The tearoom is usually found in a beautiful Japanese garden. It is sparsely furnished and may have sliding doors. Guests are dressed in traditional kimono and are greeted by their host. They remove their shoes and take their places on the mat while *kashi* (sweet candy snacks) are served. The *kama* (kettle) is put on a hot coal burner for the water to boil.

The host then brings the items to a small table to start preparing the tea which include: the tea bowl bearing a napkin, the whisk, the tea scoop and the tea caddy along with the wastewater container, the kettle's lid rest and the water ladle.

The key steps to a successful Japanese tea ceremony:

- Taking the *fukusa* (square of silk cloth) from his sash, the host wipes the tea scoop and the tea container with pure concentration and meditation. The cleansing symbolizes to the guests that everything is clean and pure. He ladles the hot water into a tea bowl, washes the tea whisk and then pours the water away. The bowl is cleaned again with the cloth and put back in its place. Now the tea can be made.

- The host puts three scoops of powdered green tea into the tea bowl, and then adds enough boiling water to the tea to make a paste, whisking it briskly. He then picks up the tea bowl and places it on top of his left palm and holds the right side of the bowl with his right hand. He turns the bowl twice away from himself with a full turn of the wrist and then places it in front of the guest who will hold it in the same way.
- The first guest turns and bows to the guest sitting next to her and offers the tea bowl. Bowing in return, this guest declines, and the first guest raises the bowl and bows in gratitude before drinking from the side of the bowl.
- She wipes off the bowl with her thumb and finger and turns the bowl back to the front, admiring the bowl and asking questions about its name and origin. The bowl is returned to the host who rinses the bowl. The whole process is then repeated for each guest.

The tea ceremony can take up to four hours. After the guests have taken tea, the host cleans the utensils and allows the guests to examine some of them. These can often be priceless antiques and a cloth is used to handle them. As the guests leave the house, the host bows from the door.

The Kimono, White Socks and Tea

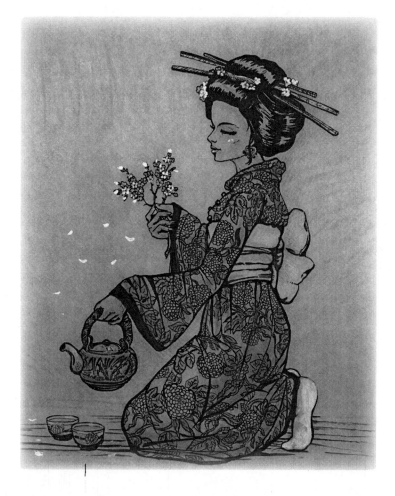

It is customary for guests and the host to wear kimonos and *tabi* (divided white toe socks). The socks allow a quieter shuffle across the mats in the tearoom while the kimono restricts stride-length. The tea ceremony takes into account the length of the host's kimono sleeves, and the motions for cleaning the tea bowl and preparing the tea. These are extremely specific in order to prevent the kimono sleeves from becoming soiled. Silk cloths for cleaning the tea bowls are folded and tucked into the sash, the *obi*.

Yak Butter Tea in Tibet -
Po Cha - For Life and Death

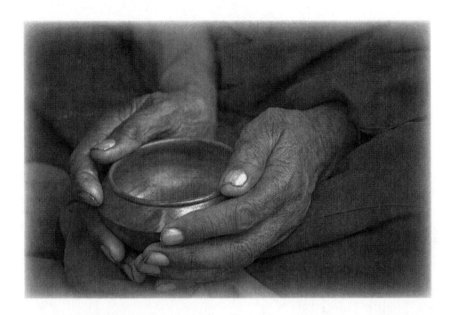

The Dalai Lama on tea:

> *"The difference between ethics and religion is like the differ-*
> *ence between water and tea. Ethics without religious content*
> *is water, a critical requirement for health and survival. Ethics*
> *grounded in religion is tea, a nutritious and aromatic blend of*
> *water, tea leaves, spices, sugar and, in Tibet, a pinch of salt.*

> *"But however the tea is prepared, the primary ingredient is al-*
> *ways water," he says. "While we can live without tea, we*
> *can't live without water. Likewise, we are born free of reli-*
> *gion, but we are not born free of the need for compassion."*

Yak butter tea is made from black tea leaves, yak butter and salt. Owing to its high caloric value, the strong buttered tea keeps the Tibetans warm and helps them maintain a good level of energy while living at such high altitudes. The tea also helps them digest the yak meat they eat three times daily, 365 times a year.

Known as *Po cha*, large quantities of tea are enjoyed throughout the day either in private homes or at teahouses before work. As a guest in a private home, it is the tradition to receive a bowl of hot butter tea and drink it in sips. After each sip, the host refills the bowl so it never becomes empty. This is the sign of a generous host.

As a guest, if you do not wish to drink the tea, it is best not to sip at all and leave the bowl full until you leave. In this way you will not offend your host.

The Nomads will often drink up to forty cups of butter tea a day, not only for energy but also to prevent chapped lips. The best buttered tea is made by leaving black tea leaves to brew in boiling water for a half a day. The tea is skimmed and poured into a churn containing fresh yak butter and salt. The tea is churned and then poured into clay teapots or jars.

Butter tea is traditionally served in wooden bowls. In private homes, two bowls are set on the main table: the larger bowl is for the man of the house, and the smaller one for his wife.

Some of the more affluent families have bowls with silver lids, which are carved with patterns to symbolize good luck. Wealthier families go further by inlaying silver throughout the bowl with only one small spot at the bottom of the bowl revealing its wooden base.

In the Tibetan world of tea, the finest tea bowl could cost you 10 yaks.

Tea trays often come in the shape of eight lotus petals with a good luck symbol engraved onto each. These represent the traditional eight propitious Tibetan symbols.

When a Tibetan dies, their wooden bowl is filled with buttered tea and placed before the corpse. On the seventh day, after the celestial burial where the dead person's body is offered to birds of prey to enable his or her spirit's flight to heaven, the family follows the funeral master to the banks of the Lhasa River. Here, the dead person's tea bowl is filled with tea to wish their spirit a safe voyage. The bowl is then cleaned and becomes the property of the funeral master. If the family chooses to keep the wooden bowl, they must buy it from the master.

Butter Tea Recipe

Ingredients

6 cups water

3 tea bags (ordinary black tea)

¼ tsp salt

2 tablespoons butter

½ cup milk or 1 tsp milk powder

Preparation

1. Boil six cups of water.
2. Put three tea bags or one heaping tablespoon of loose tea in the water and steep for two minutes.
3. Remove tea bags (or strain the tea leaves if you use loose tea).
4. Add salt, butter, and milk or milk powder into a blender or shaker with the tea.
5. Blend or shake the mixture for two to three minutes.
6. Serve immediately warm.

The Way of Moroccan Tea -
For Friendship and Respect

"The first glass is as gentle as life, the second glass
is as strong as love, the third glass is as bitter as death."
-Unknown.

Since the eighteenth century, the *Maghrebi* tea culture in Morocco has been considered an art form. *Maghreb* tea is now served throughout North Africa *(Maghreb)* and southern Spain. The British brought over green tea to the *Maghreb* in the eighteenth century and as it spread throughout the country, trade between the *Maghreb* and Europe began to flourish

Maghreb tea is made from Chinese green tea and mint leaves. It is a staple in Algeria, Morocco and Tunisia where it is served with food when guests come to visit.

It is seen as highly impolite if you refuse their offer of tea, and it is wise to accept two cups out of respect to your host. When I was in Egypt visiting the bazaars and bartering with traders, business was inevitably accompanied with mint tea to "sweeten" the edge of a deal.

As in China, Japan and Tibet, the tea tradition of good hospitality in Morocco is equally observed to guarantee you are well received by your host and as a host, respected by your guests.

Mint tea forms an essential part of a daily ritual where a skilled pouring technique is vital. Tea is poured from a height to create froth on the surface. The tradition is to pour at least three servings for each person, The tea will change in taste with each cup, depending on how long it has steeped.

⟨ ⟩ Mint Tea Recipe ⟨ ⟩

Ingredients

2 cups of water

1 tbsp of gunpowder
   green tea

1 handful of fresh
   mint leaves

2 tbsp sugar

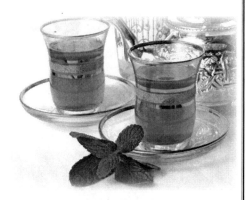

Preparation

1. Bring the water to a boil in a saucepan. Turn the heat down to simmer.

2. Rinse the gunpowder green tea leaves with boiling water to remove dust, and then add to the simmering water in the pan.

3. Add a handful of freshly picked mint leaves (or spearmint). Add sugar to taste.

4. Continue to simmer the tea, mint and sugar brew for five minutes.

5. Pour the brew through a fine meshed strainer or sieve into another pan or Moroccan tea pot with long spout. Adjust the sweetness if required.

6. Having warmed your tea glasses or cups, serve the tea from a height of about 12 inches or more into the cups to create a froth. (Tip: you can pour the tea in and out of the teapot and into the clean pan a number of times to get a good froth really going).

White "Coffee" in Beirut - Tea in Disguise

While visiting a local cookery school in Beirut, I was given the choice of coffee or "white coffee," *ahwah baida*. I opted for the latter, thinking that it would have milk and sugar.

The "white coffee" turned out not to be coffee at all; there was absolutely no trace of caffeine. Feeling a little confused, I discovered it was a delightful clean drink of rose water distilled from real roses.

"White coffee" can also be served with orange blossom infused in hot water. Both of these teas are soothing for the digestion and very refreshing. Perfect over ice on a hot summer's day.

❧ White Coffee Recipe ❧

Ingredients
1 cup of water
1 tsp of orange blossom water or rose water

Preparation
1. Pour one tsp of orange blossom water or rose water into a small cup and bring water to a boiling point
2. Add the sugar to the boiling water, reduce to a simmer.
3. Allow to cool slightly and then pour the water into the cup containing the orange blossom or rose water.

Be sure to purchase organic or true orange blossom or rose water. There are chemical variations that will not bring the same health benefits.

Tea in Russia -
The *Samovar* for Hospitality

"The little samovar slowly began to get hot, and all at once,
unexpectedly, broke into a tremulous bass hum".
- Anton Chekhov, The Dependents.

The Russians enjoy tea most of all with their co-workers and friends. It doesn't matter what cups are being used; good conversation is what matters.

A tea tip for spotting a Russian? Look at how they drink their tea. If they drink their tea with the teaspoon in the cup, they are likely to be Russian.

Russians like their black tea served in a tea glass called a *podstakannik,* which has a base made from silver or nickel silver. Like their British counterparts, they like to have their tea with something sweet, including cookies, candies, chocolate or pancakes. Many Russians drink their tea with honey or condensed milk.

The Russian *samovar* is a large metal teakettle used for heating water. It has a faucet in the middle from which to pour the hot water. The *samovar* has long been the Russian symbol of hospitality and comfort, and is often mentioned in Russian literature.

The Russians like to prepare a strong black bitter tea called *zavarka* made from dark Indian or Chinese black teas, and another favorite is the slightly smoky Russian Caravan, blended with *oolong,*

27

keemun and *souchong lapsang* teas. The tea is kept in a small teapot on top of the *samovar* and is diluted with boiling water to create a tea according to the drinker's preferred strength. Sugar, lemon, honey or jam is then added.

Today in Russia, the conversations around tea may revolve around personal issues and life in general, moving on to God and then more abstract themes. The purpose of drinking tea is to forget about everyday existence and to enjoy the art of conversation.

Tea made its treacherous journey from China to Russia around the year 1618. At first the Russians were not so keen on the taste of tea after a Chinese ambassador presented Russian Czar Michael with a chest of black tea. However, in the late 1600s, Russia and China signed a treaty and the tea trade to Russia opened up. But the journey and the incredibly taxing conditions with which the camel trains had to cross and endure for sixteen to eighteen months, put a high price on tea, and for the most part only the czar and the wealthiest families in Russia could enjoy the it.

Today, drinking tea in Russia is very much a part of social culture and an indicator of personal attitudes. If you are offered tea from yesterday, it means your Russian host wants you to leave and not outstay your welcome. If a family stops having tea together, then there is likely a problem among its members.

Spicy *Chai* in India

Chai or *massala chai* (spiced tea) originated from India about 9,000 years ago and was created by a king who drank it as an Ayurvedic cleansing drink. Originally *chai* was made from spices and didn't contain any tea leaves, and therefore was caffeine free.

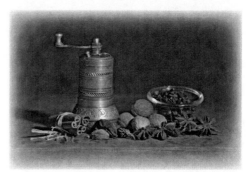

Today it is a mix of black tea with spices and milk. *Chai's* name is said to have originated from the Chinese word for tea, *cha*.

The Western term for "chai tea" is incorrect, as this translates into "tea tea." To be accurate, simply ask for a *chai*.

It wasn't until 1835, when the British first started growing black tea in Assam, that tea leaves made their way into *chai* houses. From hereon, the custom of adding milk and sweetener grew, although the drink was still not very popular because of its high cost.

However in the early 1900s, massala chai began to spread as vendors recognized the value of keeping their costs down by blending spices and milk with the black tea.

Chai wallahs are street vendors who sell tea to the public. Popular *chai* time is around 4:00 pm as tea is served with a savory snack like *samosas*, *pakoras* or *farsan*.

The spread of spiced tea to the rest of the world has seen variations on recipes, and often soy, rice or non-dairy milks are added. Green or *rooibos* tea leaves are used, instead of black, to reduce caffeine levels.

Chai Tea Ingredients

Ayurvedic philosophy and medicine consider the spices added to black tea to be *sattvic,* or calming, vitalizing and mentally clarifying.

The spices are:

Black Pepper
Widely used to support circulation and metabolism, black pepper is warming and can help to alleviate chronic coldness and warm the muscles.

Cardamom
A popular spice, it is said to benefit the lungs, kidneys, and heart. It is also a mood elevator.

Cinnamon
Believed to increase circulation and deepen breathing, increase awareness and vitality, and reduce fatigue. It is also reputed to be an aphrodisiac.

Clove
From the spice islands of Indonesia, cloves have been used by the Chinese since 300 B.C., and came to Europe in the fourth and fifth centuries A.D. Cloves have pain-relieving and antiseptic attributes. Like pepper and ginger, clove is also used to increase the potency of other herbal blends.

Fennel
An important medicinal plant in the royal herb gardens of medieval France and Germany, fennel is still widely used to treat both kidney and eye problems, as well as laryngitis.

Ginger
Invaluable for motion sickness, nausea, vomiting and stomach cramps, and helps to keep the colon clean.

Nutmeg
Nutmeg has been used for centuries to ease sciatica and promote the digestion of heavy foods. Ancient Arab physicians treated kidney and lymphatic problems with the spice.

Chinese Star Anise
It's used frequently as a cough remedy and to freshen the breath. It is also a great herb for the digestive system, calming and easing flatulence.

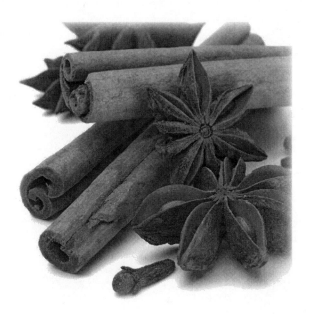

⟨ ⟩ Chai Tea Recipe ⟨ ⟩

Ingredients
⅛ tsp of each of the spices listed previously
1 tsp of loose black tea
½ cup milk
½ cup water
Sugar to taste

Preparation:
When making your *chai,* you may have a preference for a particular spice and will make that the larger portion of your spice blend.

1. Put ⅛th of a tsp from each of the spices into a mortar and grind them together. If you have included star anise, your blend will have a strong aniseed flavor.
2. Bring the milk and water to a boil then simmer.
3. Put the spices and loose black tea into the pan and allow the *chai* to simmer for about 5 mins depending on your taste buds. If you prefer something lighter, let it brew for 2 minutes.
4. Strain the tea into your cup adding sugar to taste.

The English Tea

Stands the Church clock at ten to three?
And is there honey still for tea?
Ruper Brooke, "The Old Vicarage, Grantchester" 1912

On a warm summer's afternoon in England either in a garden, a local church, a tearoom, or a cricket match; someone somewhere is sitting with a pot of tea, cakes and sandwiches, or even just a mug of tea. The tradition of the quintessential English tea has certainly changed over the centuries.

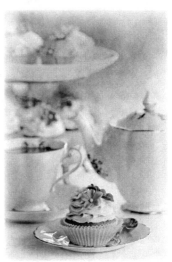

These days the grander afternoon tea affairs with their fine porcelain china, tiered cake stands brimming with fancy, delectable sweet and savory bites are more widely practiced in luxury hotels, tearooms and some of the wealthier or stately homes of England.

For most people today, a cup of tea is drunk regularly throughout the day, using the poorer quality but strong tea found in tea bags.

The "real" tea in Britain is still black tea, and the preparation of it in a teapot is still as important today as it was back in the seventeenth century when tea was first introduced.

China teapots, some say, give the tea a better flavor while metal teapots will keep the tea hotter for longer. The teapot is always warmed first with hot water and then poured away. A teaspoon. of tea per person is then added with boiling water. The tea is brewed no longer than three minutes, and then strained and served. Traditionally, milk is added to the cup first (this was initially done to stop the hot tea from cracking the cup) and then the tea is poured, with sugar added.

Black tea, often from India, will be served without milk and with a slice of lemon. For afternoon tea, *darjeeling* tea is served since it has a lighter taste compared to the stronger breakfast tea.

High tea was more of working family affair, with a heavier meal of meat and pies served with tea and eaten from a high table (compared to the lower more delicate tea tables) at around 5:00 p.m.

Tea is still very much part of the work ethic in England, and at one time many factories and large organizations would still have tea breaks at 11:00 am and 3:00 pm for their staff. I can vaguely remember the tea trolley being taken around at the BBC when I worked there. Sadly, the tradition of the tea trolley was dropped. Nobody could make tea quite like the BBC tea ladies!

Typical English Light Bites for Afternoon Tea

- Cucumber and cream cheese bite-sized sandwiches
- Smoked salmon finger sandwiches
- Egg and cress finger sandwiches, mixed with mayonnaise or Salad Cream, a popular U.K. mayonnaise brand.
- Cream cheese and dill finger sandwiches
- Welsh Rarebit- cheese melted on toast
- Scones, jam and clotted cream
- Short bread
- Tea fruit cake
- Fondant fancies

Flowering Tea – floral art for your mind, body and soul

The meditation and art behind the whole
process of tea making truly comes
into bloom when you
are able to put your tea
in a glass teapot, add hot
water, and watch as it turns
slowly, gracefully and color-
fully into an exquisite flower.

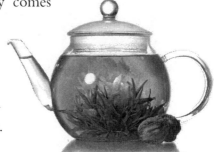

How Flower Tea is Made

These curiously simple, and at first glance, unattractive little balls
of tea are hand sewn in remote tea gardens in the southwestern
Yunnan province of China, near the borders of Laos and Vietnam.

White, green and black tea leaves are picked in the early morning and flattened, while still damp, and mixed with flowers such
as jasmine or chrysanthemum. They are then sewn with cotton
thread into various shapes and bundles. The leaves might also be
fragranced or flavored with other flower and fruit scents.

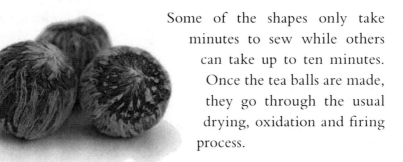

Some of the shapes only take
minutes to sew while others
can take up to ten minutes.
Once the tea balls are made,
they go through the usual
drying, oxidation and firing
process.

You can use a flowering tea two or three times once it has un-furled its leaves, but ensure you decant the tea into cups within a short period of time so that the leaves don't stay in the hot water and lose their flavor.

From the Tea Bush to your Teacup

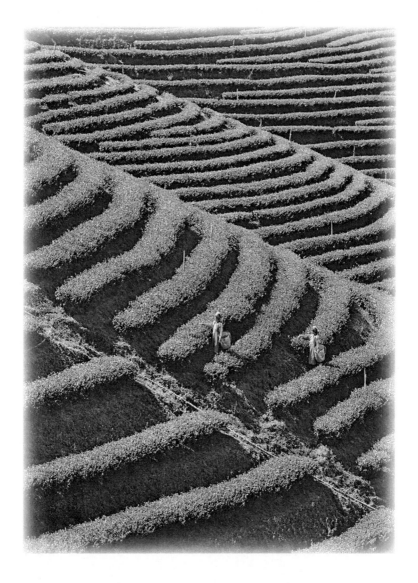

*"Strange how a teapot can represent at the same time
the comforts of solitude and the pleasures of company."*
-*Zen Haiku*

The Journey of the Humble Tea leaf

All teas whether, black, green, white or *oolong*, come from the same shrub, the *Camellia sinensis* and all of the harvested leaves start out in the same way – they are green when picked and turn brown or black the longer they are left to dry and ferment. It is the way in which the tea is processed that gives the tea its unique flavor.

The *Camellia sinensis* tea bush creates natural occurring phyto-chemicals called polyphenols that it uses for its own protection and health.

These compounds also include flavonoids that have the same health benefits as antioxidants found in fruit and vegetables. A tea shoot consists of two young leaves and a bud. At least half of it contains fiber and does not dissolve in water. The other half is soluble and contains amino acids, caffeine, sugars, vitamins and organic acids.

The tea's flavor comes from the oils in the leaves, while their tannins give the tea its astringency and color.

If you add milk and sugar to your tea and drink about six cups a day, you can expect to add 240 calories to your daily diet; so it's better to drink tea in moderation if you are watching your waistline.

The following pages outline how tea may help to improve your health.

The Tea Leaf's Journey Begins

Tea Picking: The ancient tradition of tea picking has remained fundamentally the same, with slightly varying techniques among tea producers. The tea leaf's journey from the bush to your cup is quite a process, but well worth it.

Plucking: Twice a year during late spring or early summer (occasionally Autumn or Winter), pickers pick tea leaves and flushes, which include a terminal bud and two young leaves, from the *Camellia sinensis* bush. Picking is done by hand when a higher quality tea is needed, or by a machine for a lower quality leaf.

Withering/Wilting: The tea leaves begin to wilt soon after picking. Withering removes excess water from the leaves and allows a very slight amount of oxidation. The leaves are left out in the sun or in a cool, well-ventilated room where they will lose more than a quarter of their weight in water. The process will increase the availability of freed caffeine, both of which change the taste of the tea.

Disruption: or "leaf maceration" is where the teas are bruised or torn in order to promote and quicken oxidation. The leaves can also be lightly bruised on their edges by shaking and tossing them in a bamboo tray or tumbling in baskets. Machines can also be used to do the tearing and crushing and this makes the leaves release more juices and commence their oxidation.

Oxidation/Fermentation: Some teas will require longer oxidation, depending on the final taste required by the producer. These leaves are left in a climate-controlled environment and will turn progressively darker. The chlorophyll breaks down and tannins are released. This process is fundamental in the formation of the tea's taste and fragrance.

Fixation/Kill-green: Kill-green or "shaqing" is controlling the tea leaves' oxidation level. They are either steamed or panned in a wok. For some white and black teas such as CTC (crush, tear and curl) teas, kill-green is done simultaneously while drying the leaves.

Sweltering/Yellowing: This process takes the leaves from the previous stage and heats them lightly, turning the green leaves to a yellow color, giving them a brisk and mellow taste.

Rolling/Shaping: The tea leaves are now ready to be rolled or shaped by hand or machine. The rolling action helps to further disperse any essential oils or juices left inside the leaves.

Drying: To get the tea ready for sale, it needs to be dried and is often baked, taking care not to overcook the leaves for risk of losing their flavor.

Aging/Curing: Once the baking is done, some teas will require additional aging or more fermentation. *Pu'erh* tea is often bitter and needs further curing while *oolong tea* will improve if it is fired over charcoal. For flavored teas, the manufacturer will spray the tea with fragrances or store them with flavoring essences or flowers such as jasmine.

Grading Tea Leaves

Tea leaves are graded so tea experts can evaluate and compare different varieties of tea and assess their monetary value. The grading is primarily undertaken for black tea only.

The grading of green tea and *oolong* tea differs from that of black tea. Green tea is graded by the variety of the tea plant; its taste, its origin, the climate it was cultivated in; the time the leaves were picked, and whether it is made of whole leaves (which is a good sign).

Black tea is graded on mainly two factors:

1. Size. Whole, larger tea leaves receive higher grading.

2. Production method. The methods are either by hand or machine, the latter known as CTC (crush, tear and curl). Mechanized methods can damage the tea leaves, creating a lower grade of tea.

The grades of Black tea are:

Dust D – an inferior grade of tea, which contains small pieces of tea leaves and tea dust.

Fanning – a lower grade that consists of small pieces of tea leaves.

BOP – Broken Orange Pekoe – this is a medium grade of tea consisting of both small and large leaves.

OP – Orange Pekoe – a higher grading of tea where the large, whole tea leaves are picked without the flower bud of the tea plant.

FOP – Flowery Orange Pekoe –a high grade tea where whole tea leaves are combined with the flowering tea bud.

Golden hues in the tea leaves combined with an abundance of young tea buds (referred to as "tippy") are signs of a very high quality tea.

The word pekoe describes the white hairs on the side of the tea leaves. The term means small, whole leaf tea.

The Best Quality Tea:

GFOP – Golden Flowery Orange Pekoe – young whole leaves, golden tips.

TGFOP – Tippy Golden Flowery Orange Pekoe – combines tea buds and two uppermost leaves of the tea plant. This category is the highest grade of tea leaves and is further broken down into: Fine Tippy Golden Flowery Orange Pekoe and Super Fine.

Tea Tasting

The art of tea tasting is very similar to wine tasting and the tea experts put themselves through a variety of sensory tests to demonstrate their skills as

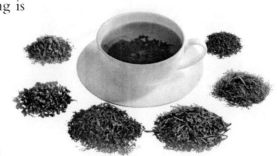

they taste, smell, and feel the tea leaves; checking their shape, size and color.

This sensory test is still the most widely accepted method of evaluating the quality of the tea and involves the tea tasters sitting around a large table with bowls of dry tea leaves for them to inspect before the tea is brewed.

The tea leaves are weighed for brewing before hot water is added. Brewing takes up to 6 minutes then the tea is poured for tasting and the tea leaves removed for inspection.

The different teas are tasted with a teaspoon, similar to wine tasting, the taster moves the tea through his mouth to gain the best impression of the tea. The taster then spits the tea into a spittoon and moves on to the next tea.

No milk or sugar is added unless it is a tasting for the British market so that they can ascertain whether the tea works with milk.

Tea experts have their own vocabulary when it comes to describing tea. Some of these you may want to use to impress your friends. There are many but here are a few selected phrases:

The agony of the leaves: The agony of it all! The longer your tea leaves take to unfurl while steeping in hot water, the longer the agony of the leaf and the better the tea tastes. At this point, this whole process seems quite mean!

Astringency: Teas rich in polyphenols (antioxidants) will create a tingling sensation in the mouth, hence the astringency.

Bakey: If the tea has been dried at too high a temperature, the leaves will smell as if they have been baked.

Body: This is the strength of taste and fullness of flavor as the tea tickles your taste buds.

Bright: A good sign if the tea leaves a tingly sensation in your mouth and feel light.

Flat: The tea has a poor taste and is of low quality. This can also indicate a tea past its prime or its poor storage. "Musty" is also another term for tea with a moldy taste.

Smooth: The tea has a silky pleasant taste.

Tea versus Coffee in the Caffeine Stakes

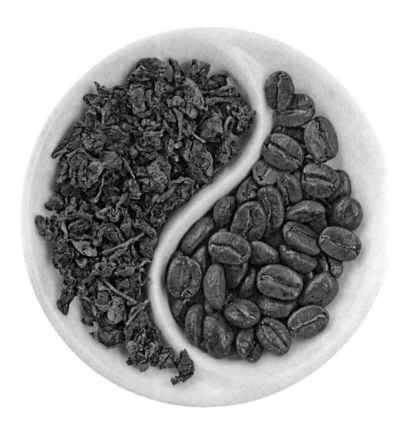

*"If this is coffee, please bring me some tea; but if
this is tea, please bring me some coffee."*
- Abraham Lincoln

Caffeine

According to the Mayo Clinic, an 8 fl oz serving of generic brewed coffee contains 95-200 mg of caffeine while the same size cup of decaffeinated coffee has about 2-12 mg of caffeine.

On average, caffeine in tea is about half that of coffee. The recommended daily dosage of caffeine is 200-300 mg per day, about two to three cups maximum, but you need to watch out for any health issues. The Mayo Clinic suggests that if a person experiences irritability, restlessness, an upset stomach, heart palpitations, or insomnia after drinking coffee or tea, he or she should either cut back or stop caffeine completely.

What is Caffeine?

Caffeine is a naturally occurring chemical stimulant called trimethylxanthine and is a drug to stimulate brain function and focus.

Tea contains tannins which slow down the absorption of caffeine in the blood. Tannins are released over an extended period of time so they actually prevent a caffeine high and a subsequent crash in energy. Caffeine in coffee, unfortunately, enters your bloodstream immediately, gives you a buzz and then brings you crashing down.

Brewing times for your tea will affect the amount of caffeine released into your cup.

Whether you are choosing, black, *oolong, pu'erh,* green or white tea, each holds a certain amount of caffeine. The length of time you brew your chosen tea will determine how much caffeine is released in your drink.

For example, if you pour boiling water on your barely caffeinated white tea and allow it to steep for six minutes, your white tea could end up with nearly as much caffeine as black tea.

If you brew the white tea at a lower water temperature and let it steep for one to two minutes, there will be minimal caffeine content.

Caffeine depends on the tea grade and whether the tea leaves are twisted or rolled.

If you choose a high quality tea made from brand new tips or buds of the tea plant, it will have more antioxidants and nutrients than tea made from the same plant's older leaves. However, it will also bear more caffeine.

If you are using loose tea, observe the shape of the leaves. If they are rolled or twisted, the caffeine may release more slowly into the brew than from flat or open leaves.

Blended teas have less caffeine.

When you purchase a blended loose black tea with herbs and fruits, you will use the same amount of water for brewing one teaspoon of tea. Since there are fewer tea leaves and more fruits and herbs, there will be less caffeine in your drink compared to a cup of black tea.

Powdered Green Tea and Caffeine

Matcha green tea is ground into a fine powder from the entire tea leaf, giving it a higher level of caffeine compared to the infusion of tea leaves in hot water. *Matcha* tea plants are grown in the shade, increasing their caffeine content. When a tea bush is restricted of sunlight, the amount of chlorophyll and other chemical compounds, including caffeine, increase in the leaves.

Methods for Decaffeinating Tea

Decaffeinated tea contains a small percentage of caffeine, but less than the average caffeinated cup. When you purchase decaffeinated tea, one of the following organic solvents may have been used to extract its caffeine.

Methylene chloride: Tea leaves are soaked in this solvent, which absorbs the caffeine. This is then re-poured over the tea to add flavor and fragrance. The U.S. has banned all imports using methylene chloride, the same chemical found in paint strippers, aerosol sprays and dry cleaning solutions.

Ethyl acetate: This is a naturally occurring chemical found in tea leaves. Caffeine is extracted in the same way as with the methylene chloride process. However, ethyl acetate is very difficult to remove after the decaffeination process, and can leave a chemical taste.

Carbon dioxide (CO2): Pressurized carbon dioxide liquefies and acts as the most preferred solvent to extract caffeine from tea leaves. In this process, moistened leaves are exposed to the pressurized CO2. After some hours, the liquid is poured out and the leaves are dried. CO2 decaffeinated teas best retain the original flavors of the tea.

Water: Primarily used for coffee decaffeination. Caffeine is extracted from the tea leaves by soaking them in hot water for a period of time. The liquid is then passed through a carbon filter to strain out the caffeine. The water is then returned to the tea leaves for a reabsorption of flavors and oils. Flavors can be lost during this process, resulting in a weaker tea.

The CO 2 process is considered the best method for decaffeinating tea.

Try this simple washing technique at home to decaffeinate your tea

Fill half a teapot with boiling water containing a tea bag or tea leaves. Allow the tea to steep for about twenty seconds, and then drain it. Add more hot water and repeat the process two to three times. By the fourth round, the flavor will grow more intense and your tea will be virtually caffeine-free.

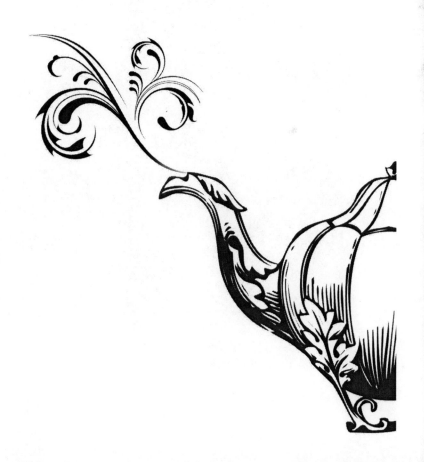

The Wisdom of Drinking
the Humble Tea leaf
The Health Benefits of Tea

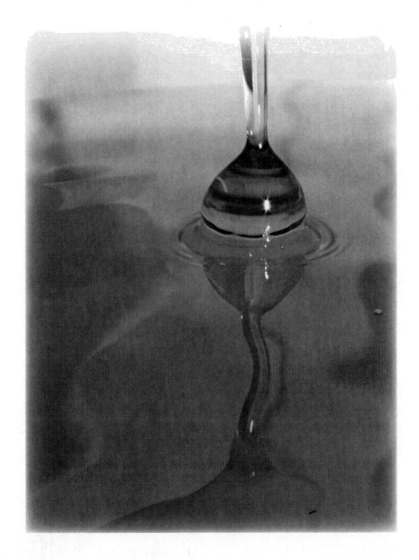

"If people drank a cup of tea everyday, the pharmacists would starve."
- Chinese proverb

Black Tea – for mental alertness and a healthy heart

Black tea is the most oxidized tea available and contains about 40–60 mg of caffeine per 8 fl oz cup, whereas decaffeinated tea has 0–12 mg per cup. Black tea is stronger in flavor and more robust compared to green or white tea.

According to the U.S. Agriculture Research Services' Diet and Human Laboratory, about 75 percent of the tea produced worldwide is black tea.

Generally, unblended black teas are named after the region in which they were produced. Here are just some of the more well-known varieties:

- *Tanyang Gongfu* – the leader of the *Fujian* artisan red teas and grown in the Fujian Province, it has a mild sweet potato taste.
- *Lapsang souchong* – the leaves are dried over burning pine, giving a strong smoky flavor. Grown in the Fujian Province.

- *Keemun* – one of China's famous teas, which is fruity with hints of pine.
- *Assam* – the most produced tea in the world, it has a full bodied malty taste. Grown along the banks of the Brahmaputra River in northeastern India, Assam is an ideal breakfast tea. It is the main tea leaf used for blending with other teas, including English Breakfast Tea.
- *Darjeeling* – floral and fruity with a unique spice, it can often be a blend of *oolong*, green and black tea leaves and is considered to be the highest quality and tastiest of black teas available. The tea bushes grow on the high, steep slopes of the Himalayan Mountains and benefit from sunshine, cooler temperatures at night and rainfall. A slight tingling sensation on the tongue is the sign of a good quality *Darjeeling*.
- *Ceylon* – grown on elevated plantations in Sri Lanka, this tea is honey golden in color and light. Teas grown on lower plantations are stronger and burgundy brown in color.

Blended Black Teas

It was during the Ming Dynasty when Chinese tea drinkers began adding fruits and fragrances to their teas and also discovered that tea leaves are extremely absorbent and will easily take on the fragrance of fresh flowers. Some examples of these fragrant teas are:

- Earl Grey – blended with bergamot, a small tart orange. Tea leaves are flavored with the oil to give a fragrant light taste. The tea is named after British Prime Minister Earl Charles Grey (1830-1834) who was given the gift of bergamot tea from a Chinese envoy. This tea was one of the first teas to be produced and gained a place of honor with the British nobility. Twinings of London claim to have the original recipe for the tea as do Jackson's of Piccadilly.

- English Breakfast —is a combination of Assam, Ceylon and Kenyan tea leaves to go with milk and sugar.
- Irish Breakfast – is blended with several black teas.
- *Masala Chai* —blends black tea leaves with spices, sugar or honey.

Recipes are given on page 122 for blending your own black teas with essential oils and becoming the timeless tea artisan.

The Health Benefits of Black Tea

Black tea is rich in antioxidants and vital minerals such as calcium, manganese, copper, selenium and potassium as well as vitamins A, B, C, E and K, and folic acids, niacinamide, and other detoxifying alkaloids.

Research shows that if you drink black tea (without milk) daily, it may help:

- **As an antioxidant** - according to the Central Food Technological Research Institute in Mysore, India, their extensive research concludes that black tea possesses free radical-scavenging and metal-chelating abilities.
- **Be effective against inflammation and several types of cancer**.
- **Reduce DNA damage** - due to oxidative stress.
- **Prevent cardiovascular disease**.
- **Help keep weight off** - the flavonoids in black tea are powerful antioxidants which help block starches from being absorbed into your body.

- **Balance blood sugar** – according to Ernst J. Schaefer of HNRCA's Lipid Metabolism Laboratory, blood sugar levels could be lowered by 15-20 percent after drinking six cups of black tea per day for eight weeks.
- **Reduce the risk of coronary heart disease** – a six to ten percent reduction in blood lipids can be achieved in three weeks by drinking five servings of black tea daily.

Medline Plus is a service of the U.S. National Library of Medicine and offers some valuable information on the benefits of black tea:

- **Mental alertness**. Drinking black tea and other caffeinated beverages throughout the day helps to keep people alert, even after extended periods without sleep.
- **Prevents dizziness** upon standing up (orthostatic hypotension) in older people. Black tea works for this condition because it raises blood pressure.
- **Reduces the risk of heart attacks**. There is some evidence that people who drink black tea have a lower risk of a heart attack. If they do have a heart attack, they are less likely to die if they have been drinking black tea for at least a year.
- **Reduces the risk of kidney stones**. Women who drink black tea appear to have an eight percent lower risk of developing kidney stones.
- **Reduces the risk of ovarian cancer**. Women who regularly drink tea, including black tea or green tea, appear to have a significantly lowered risk of developing ovarian cancer compared to women who never or seldom drink tea.
- **Reduces the risk of hardening of the arteries** (atherosclerosis), especially in women.

Avoid: As with all caffeine drinks, avoid black tea if you are pregnant, suffer from anxiety, irritable bowel syndrome, diarrhea, or high blood pressure. If you have osteoporosis, minimize the number of cups you have per day, since caffeine can leach calcium, and possibly iron from the body.

Pu'erh Tea – To aid digestion and reduce the effects of alcohol

Pu'erh tea is stronger than black tea, and comes from the county of Pu'erh in the Yunnan Province of China. *Pu'erh* contains about 60-70 mg of caffeine per 8 fl oz cup. The taste is very smooth and the longer you keep the tea in storage, the better it tastes.

Pu'erh tea can be traced back to the Han Dynasty (202 B.C.E.-220 C.E.) and is made from the leaves of the *da ye* or broad leaf tea bush. The leaves are put through a delicate maturation process creating *maocha* which means "rough tea."

Tea cakes known as "raw green *pu'erh"* are pressed from the "rough tea."

The tea is put through an artificial aging process for forty days which creates a bacterial and fungal microflora that gives the tea its widely known medicinal benefits. After fermentation, the tea is dried, pressed and classified as cooked/black *pu'erh*.

Traditionally, the tea was always pressed raw and vaulted up to 100 years to gain the best fermentation. Aged *pu'erh* tea is mellow and leaves a sweet taste in the mouth.

According to the Web MD website:

"There is interest in using pu'erh tea for lowering cholesterol because, unlike other teas, it contains small amounts of a chemical called lovastatin. Lovastatin is a prescription medicine used for lowering cholesterol. Investigators believe that the bacteria contaminating pu-erh tea may somehow make the lovastatin compound in the course of their normal life cycle. Animal research suggests that pu-erh tea might lower certain blood fats called triglycerides as well as total and "bad" low-density lipoprotein (LDL) cholesterol. It might also raise "good" high density lipoprotein (HDL) cholesterol."

The Health Benefits of Pu'erh Tea

Pu'erh tea has long been revered throughout Asia for its medicinal benefits. It may help:

- **Digestion** - to cut through grease and cholesterol, and to aid digestion after meals.
- **Warms** - if feeling chilled or at the onset of a cold.
- **Alcohol** - reduces the effects of alcohol and a hangover.
- **Stimulate the mind**.
- **Blood pressure and cholesterol** - better than green tea for lowering triglycerides, blood pressure and cholesterol levels in the body.
- **Chinese medicine** - used to inhibit internal dampness and to invigorate the activity of the spleen and stomach.
- **De-tox the body**.
- **Eyesight** - improves vision.
- **Blood Circulation** - improves blood circulation.

- **Anti-aging** – has anti-cancerous properties by attacking free radicals in the body and protecting connective tissue from damage.

Purchasing *Pu'erh* Tea

When purchasing *Pu'erh* tea, it's important to find a reputable seller from the Yunnan province of China. The packaging must state that the tea was cultivated from a wild *da ye* or broad leaf tea bush.

Also look at the price. The older the tea, the better it is, and the more expensive it will be.

Oolong Tea – for weight loss, skin disorders and easy breathing

Oolong (Black dragon) teas are semi–oxidized, making them a little bolder and more complex than green tea but not as strong as black tea. The caffeine content and antioxidant level is also mid–way between that of green and black teas, making them healthier and more palatable.

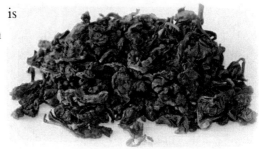

Oolong is a great favorite and popular tea with connoisseurs, especially the top grades of high mountain *oolong* from Taiwan. According to the U.S. Agriculture Research Services' Diet and Human Laboratory, about two percent of the tea produced worldwide is *oolong*.

Black Dragon Tea

All *oolong* teas come from China with many varietals having their own distinct flavors and fragrances. When *oolong* tea was first cultivated in the Wu Yi mountains of China, planters noticed that a black snake liked to make its home in the tea bush. Since snakes are known as "little dragons" in Chinese, the tea derived its name from "black dragon," pronounced "oo-lung". There is also a special category of *oolong* leaves which are minimally oxidized but rich in antioxidants, called *pouchongs*.

The tea leaves are picked and left to wither and then rolled, often by hand. The leaves are allowed to partially oxidize and then are fired in a pan or basket to arrest the oxidation process. Oxidation may range from 12–85 percent. Sometimes, charcoal smoke is used to add flavor to the tea.

Monkey Picked *Oolong* Tea

A cute name, it denotes a high quality top-of-the-line *oolong* tea. This supreme *Ti Kwan Yin olong* tea comes from the Fujian Province in China and legend has it that the Buddhist monks would train monkeys to pick the youngest leaves from the topmost branches of the rare wild tea bushes growing on the mountainside.

Today monkeys are no longer employed, but the art of plucking the freshest unbroken and evenly shaped leaves from these bushes makes this tea the highest quality of *oolong* in the world.

The Health Benefits of *Oolong* Tea

According to the USA Tea Association, *oolong,* a semi-green fermented tea, offers the same health benefits as green or black tea.

Oolong tea is rich in naturally occurring phenolic compounds. These compounds help our bodies fight oxidative damage diseases (coronary heart disease, stroke and cancers).

It may help:

- **Your immune system** – *oolong* contains polyphenols and catechins, which are powerful antioxidants. These will eliminate toxins in the body known as free radicals, which can cause premature degeneration of the internal organs. Daily use of the tea may protect against cancer since the tea has a strong alkalizing effect on excessive acidity in the body associated with cancer.
- **Skin Disorders** – according to scientific research, patients diagnosed with eczema can benefit from drinking three cups of *oolong* tea, three times a day. The beneficial results of *oolong* tea may be evident in less than a week, with some patients showing remarkable skin improvement.
- **Bone Structure** – the antioxidants present in *oolong* tea may protect against tooth decay and strengthen bone structure by reducing blood and tissue acidity, which is the primary loss of calcium from bones and teeth, or osteoporosis.
- **Type 2 Diabetes** - *oolong* tea may be effective for treating diabetic disorders according to the Research Center in Osaka, Japan. See bibliography for more information.
- **Improve water retention** - the tea has mild diuretic properties to facilitate the elimination of toxins and acids,

which are flushed from the blood and tissues through the kidneys.

- **Stress** – in a detailed study conducted at the Osaka Institute for Health Care Science in Japan, lab mice that were given *oolong* tea showed a remarkable improvement in stress levels by more than ten to eighteen percent. The natural polyphenols in the tea are said to be primary stress reducers.
- **Control Obesity** – the polyphenol compound found in *oolong* tea is very effective at controlling the fat metabolism of the body. *Oolong* drank twice daily activates certain enzymes and enhances the functions of fat cells in the human body.
- **Weight Loss:** The Chinese have long believed that *oolong* tea is beneficial in reducing and maintaining weight. Physiologist Dr. William Rumpler, of the U.S. Agriculture Research Services' Diet and Human Laboratory, investigated the ancient Chinese belief that *oolong* tea is effective in controlling body weight.

The results showed:

"Participants burned an average of 67 more calories per day when drinking the full strength oolong tea, and increased fat oxidation (fat burning) by 12 percent after consuming the full strength oolong tea for two hours."

Mountain Oolong Tea for Easy Breathing

High mountain *oolong* tea in Chinese medicine ·has long been known to detoxify and benefit digestive issues and in Japan, mountain *oolong* is used for its powerful cleansing and protective properties for the lungs. According to the *Oolong* Tea Organization, the tea works in the following way.

"… Gases suspended within the fluid of the tea are excreted from the bloodstream through the lungs, and as they pass through the delicate lung tissues with each breath, they dislodge heavy metals, tars, and other toxic residues from the air sacs and bronchia, allowing the toxins to be coughed up and spit out.

As a result of this discovery, high mountain oolong has become the beverage of choice for millions of Chinese and Japanese people, who rank among the world's heaviest smokers. Studies have shown that smokers who drink this tea throughout the day have significantly lower rates of lung cancer, emphysema, and other respiratory ailments than those who don't."

Green Tea – for a stronger immune system, radiant skin, a healthy heart and weight loss

Green tea is one of the least oxidized teas available on the market, and contains a minimal amount of caffeine, far less than black tea, but it still holds approximately 25 mg of caffeine per 8 fl oz if you brew it for longer than three minutes.

Originally from China, green tea is a legend in its own right. It has been popular both as a drink and for its medicinal properties in China for at least 4,000 years. As early as 600 and 900 A.D. the use of green tea was already being explored by Lu Yu, author of *The Tea Classic.*

According to the U.S. Agriculture Research Services' Diet and Human Laboratory, about 23 percent of the tea produced worldwide is green tea.

The polyphenols and antioxidants in green tea provide its numerous health benefits while its L-theanine content calms the nerves.

The tea plants are either grown in the shade or sun, and each growing method will alter the taste of the final tea.

Once harvested, the leaves are steamed or pan-fried to help them reach their proper color; maintain the quality of the polyphenols; and to release their aroma. The leaves are rolled tight to help the drying process and to break up the leaf tissue so that the quality of the leaf improves upon brewing.

The leaves are then dried, which brings out yet another flavor and improves their appearance.

Varieties of Green tea

There are many varieties grown both in China, Japan, Vietnam and Indonesia. The green tea plants are harvested three times a year, and it is the first flush in the spring that brings the best quality leaves.

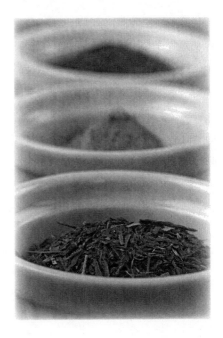

- **Gyokuro green tea** - is the finest Japanese green tea and the tea bushes are shaded from the sun for several weeks. This makes the tea grow more slowly, taking time to develop depth and flavor. The sun-deprived leaves are higher in chlorophyll, which creates the vivid green color in the leaves.

- **Sencha green tea** - comes from the first flush of the year; is known as the new tea and is one of the most popular green teas in Japan.
- **Bancha green tea** - is the lowest grade of tea and is harvested from the second flush of the *sencha*.
- **Gunpowder green tea** - is a form of green Chinese tea where each leaf is rolled into a small round ball. Its name comes from the fact that it resembles gunpowder used for rifles and cannons. It dates back to the Tang Dynasty (618 – 907 C.E.). When you purchase it, make sure that the small green balls of tea are shiny (a sign of freshness) and not dry. Small, tightly rolled pellets taste better.

The Difference between Japanese and Chinese Green Teas

The Chinese green teas are pan-fired or "roasted" during processing; the Japanese green teas are steamed for about 15 – 20 seconds to prevent the leaves from oxidizing. The steaming also gives a difference in flavor, making the Japanese green tea more grassy and bitter, but greener in color.

Powdered Green Tea *Matcha* for focus and relaxation

A Japanese favorite, matcha is made by grinding the full tea leaves into a fine powder and is prepared in a singular way, using a whisk. The Chinese and Zen Buddhists have been using *matcha* green tea for centuries to relax during meditation for three to six hours in one sitting at a time. *Matcha* helps to focus the mind and relax simultaneously, and is also noted to help us tap into deeply creative states, and sustain concentration.

Research shows that there are 137 times higher amounts of EGCGs (Epigallocatechin gallates) in *matcha* tea than green tea owing to the way in which the tea is grown and prepared. The L-theanine content is very high in this tea. L-theanine has been shown to put the brain into an alpha state, a relaxed brain wave state which brings about feelings of happiness, relaxation and well-being.

L-theanine also helps to balance caffeine and allow it to be absorbed more slowly into the body.

EGCGs give green tea its antioxidants and anti-inflammatory abilities, and when combined with caffeine will stimulate a significant reduction in body weight through thermogenesis (the body's ability to burn calories for long periods of time).
See teas for weight loss further on in the book.

Interestingly, one cup of *matcha* tea is the equivalent of ten cups of green tea in terms of antioxidant content.

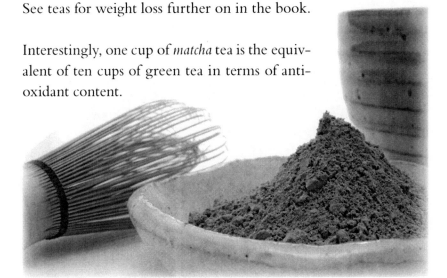

Recipe for *Usucha Matcha* (thin matcha)

To make one bowl or cup of *matcha* you will need:

Ingredients

1.5 tsp organic powdered matcha
2.5 fl oz of hot water
A clean tea cloth (*chakin*)
A pretty *matcha* bowl (*chawan*)
A bamboo *matcha* whisk (*chasen*)
A bamboo *matcha* scoop (*chashaku*)
Dairy or non-dairy milk, sweetener

Preparation

1. Fill the bowl with hot water and let it stand.
2. Stand the bamboo whisk in the bowl. Once the bowl has warmed up, throw away the water, put the whisk to one side, and wipe the bowl dry.
3. Pour hot water into a measuring jug and let it cool slightly.
4. Measure the *matcha* and place in the bowl.
5. Pour slightly cooled water over the matcha tea, and whisk rapidly with the *chasen* until tea dissolves, and liquid has a light-colored foam on the surface. The key is to use your wrist, not your arm, in whisking, making a zigzag motion in the liquid until the bubbles begin to froth.
6. *Matcha* is usually taken without sweetener or milk, but you may add soy, rice, almond or dairy milk with honey to suit your taste.

The Health Benefits of Green tea

While research continues to confirm the health benefits of green tea, science over the years has also shown that the tea's active ingredient, catechin, can outperform vitamin C in terms of scavenging free radicals from the body. In addition, its polyphenols are also more potent than vitamin C, vitamin E, rosemary extract and other antioxidants.

EGCG (Epigallocatechin gallate), found in green tea, is a catechin (a potent antioxidant) and inhibits the aging process of tissue and reduces inflammation. The anti–inflammatory properties of EGCG not only boost the immune system, but also contribute to acne-free radiant skin.

In China, the rate of cancer is lower than in other countries, and many believe it is the high rate of green tea consumption that plays a vital role in the prevention of cancer. In traditional Chinese medicine, green tea is used as as a diuretic as well as to control bleeding and prevent heart disease.

The polyphenols found in green tea have also been shown to prevent inflammation, protect cartilage, fight HPV infections, and reduce the growth of abnormal cells in the cervix, according to Medline Plus.

At the back of this book you will find numerous references to studies on green tea in addition to those below. In general, it would seem that current laboratory studies show the positive health effects of green tea, but human clinical evidence is still limited, and future research is required to further define the extent of green tea's health benefits.

Drinking green tea two or three times a day, according to Medline Plus, may also help:

- **Increase mental alertness** – due to its caffeine content.
- **Prevent dizziness** – upon standing up (orthostatic hypotension) in older people.
- **Prevent cancers** – bladder esophageal, ovarian, and pancreatic cancers. In one study, women who drank two or more cups of green tea each day had a 46 percent lower risk of getting ovarian cancer than women who didn't drink the tea.
- **Reduce the risk or delay the onset of Parkinson's disease** – drinking one to four cups of green tea daily seems to provide the most protection against developing Parkinson's.
- **Lower blood pressure** – green tea may especially help elderly people who experience low blood pressure after eating.
- **Decrease high levels of fat** – cholesterol and triglycerides.
- **Diarrhea and Typhoid** – in Asia, green tea has been used since ancient times to treat these two health issues.

Research also indicates green tea for:

- **Weight loss** – taking a specific green tea extract (EGCG) appears to help moderately overweight people lose weight. Green tea contains caffeine and EGCG, both of which help ramp up metabolism, and slow down the body's ability to store sugars and fat. This combination may increase fat oxidation, reducing your body mass index and waistline. However, keep in mind it's still important to keep to a low-fat diet and exercise in addition to drinking three cups a day. If you feel tremors, confusion, irregular or rapid heartbeat, headaches or sleep issues after drinking green tea, then stop and see your regular health care provider.

- **High blood pressure** - some research indicates that drinking green tea regularly may prevent the onset of high blood pressure. But not all studies concur.
- **Stroke prevention** - according to a large study done in Japan, drinking three cups of green tea per day seems to significantly lower the risk of having a stroke, compared to drinking one cup or no tea. Women appeared to benefit more than men.
- **Weak bones (osteoporosis)** - population research suggests that drinking green tea for 10 years is associated with stronger bones.
- **Diabetes, Type 2** - drinking green tea may help prevent diabetes. Research in Japan suggests that adults who drink six or more cups of green tea per day have a 33 percent lower risk of developing Diabetes, Type 2 compared to those who drink one cup per day or less. This is especially true for women.
- **Breast cancer** - green tea does not seem to prevent breast cancer in Asian populations. However, in Asian-American populations, some evidence suggests that drinking green tea might reduce the risk of developing breast cancer. Most research on green tea for breast cancer has been with Asian populations, therefore its effect on breast cancer among western subjects are less conclusive.
- **Gum disease** (gingivitis) - chewing candy that contains green tea extract seems to control the plaque build-up on teeth and reduce gum swelling.
- **Prostate cancer** - Chinese men who drink green tea appear to have a lower risk of developing prostate cancer.

Green tea may also positively affect the following:

- Cervical cancer.
- Dental cavities.
- Gastric cancer.
- Heart disease.
- Kidney stones.
- Leukemia.
- Lung cancer.
- Skin cancer.
- Stomach cancer.

Avoid Green tea if you are taking aspirin, warfarin or antibiotics. If you have iron-deficiency anemia, reduce your intake of green tea since it may reduce iron absorption. Allergic reactions may occur. As always, make sure to consult your health care provider.

Forever Young – Green Tea's Anti-aging Abilities

Asians appear to have long life spans and youthful skins. This may in part be attributed to the high amount of green tea they drink, which contains potent anti-aging properties, including anti-colla-genase and anti-elastase, and of course having good genes comes into play!

Collagen is a protein found in the connective tissues of the body and is important to keep the skin strong. Elastin supports the body's natural elasticity, helping the lungs, arteries, ligaments and skin to function.

Green tea can prevent enzymes from breaking down the elastin and collagen in our bodies. It can also play a role in protecting our skin from the sun. Using a green tea extract in your sunscreen (only use zinc oxide-based sunscreens; they are less likely to react with the green tea extract) may help to further protect your skin from the sun's damaging rays.

You will find some green tea recipes later in the book for anti-aging and for maintaining a healthy skin tone.

White Tea – for lowering cholesterol and reducing inflammation

White tea is a treasure of a tea made from the youngest and most tender hand-picked leaf tips and buds harvested in the spring.

Compared to green tea, white tea is very lightly oxidized and contains the fullest nutrients of the plant with minimal caffeine.

White tea first appeared in the Northern Song Dynasty (960 – 1127) when Emperor Huizong wrote a book with very specific instructions for the making and tasting of the tea.

The tea gets its name from the silvery white hairs on the unopened buds of the tea bush. White tea is mainly produced in the Jianyang, Fuding and Songxi counties in the Fujian Province of China

Varieties of White Tea

The most popular types of white tea are White Peony and Silver Needle.

White Peony gets its name from the way in which the leaves bloom like the buds of the first flowers in springtime.

The exotic Silver Needle, the most expensive of the white teas, is made only from the single tip of the tea stem, which when dried look like silver needles.

The key to making a good white tea is in the withering stage of preparation. Once the leaves have been picked, they are left to wither outdoors and then brought indoors. The process then follows very much the same as for green tea.

The Health Benefits of White Tea

In traditional Chinese medicine, white tea is highly regarded for its ability to: reduce inflammation in rheumatoid arthritis; control insulin secretion; prevent dry eyes and night blindness; reduce radiation levels, and repair DNA damage. In addition it is also known to help:

- **Anti-aging**- as with green tea, white tea is well known for its anti-aging properties due to its high levels of anti-collagenase and anti-elastase.
- **Blood Pressure** - white tea may decrease blood pressure and improve the function of blood vessels, thus decreasing the risk of cardiovascular disease.
- **Cholesterol** - white tea has been found to reduce cholesterol, owing to the catechins, a group of polyphenol antioxidants.
- **Strep and Staph Infections** - a study in 2004 at Pace University revealed that white tea extract may help slow

viruses and bacterial growth, and destroy 80 percent of viruses within ten minutes.

- **Inflammation** – a study by the School of Life Sciences at Kingston University in Southwest London revealed that white tea could reduce the risks of inflammation, a precursor to rheumatoid arthritis and some cancers.

Yellow Tea – savored and valued for its rarity

A beautiful rare Chinese tea, yellow tea has not been as widely studied as green tea and unfortunately, is more difficult and costly to produce than white or green tea.

Yellow tea is very lightly oxidized and does not have the grassy scent of green tea. It contains very little caffeine.

Varieties of Yellow Tea

At one time there were many hundreds of varieties, but owing to difficult growing locations and processing, only three varieties exist:

- *Mo Gan Huang Ya* Tea
  Prized for its delicate flavor and aroma, this tea is grown in high elevations; it is the rarest of yellow teas.

- *Meng Ding Huang Ya* Tea
  A yellow tea made famous before the Tang dynasty, it would be sent to the Imperial Palace once a year to announce the arrival of spring.

- *Junshan Yinzhen*
  Favorable growing conditions on mist-covered mountains
  give the tea its flavor and aroma. It has been a favorite
  with Chinese leaders, including the late Chairman Mao
  Zedong.

Yellow tea is harvested in the spring when the leaves are still in
bud form and have the highest amount of anti-oxidants. The
leaves are allowed to sit and yellow, which gives the tea its name.
The buds are fried to stop oxidation and then wrapped in special
paper and stored in wooden boxes. Periodically, the tea is refried
and rewrapped in paper; the process takes about three days. The
leaves are then slowly roasted.

The Health Benefits of Yellow Tea

Since these teas are so rare and specialized, they are consumed by
connoisseurs who are more interested in their taste and flavor. As
a result, there has been scant scientific evidence on their health
benefits.

However, since the processing of yellow tea is similar to that of
green tea and the leaves are picked at bud stage, its health benefits
will most likely be similar to those of green and white tea.

The tea appears to be much easier on the stomach than other teas
and now, because of its rarity, people are becoming more intrigued
by it. Demand for it has been steadily rising.

The Ritual of Tea – Making the Perfect Cup

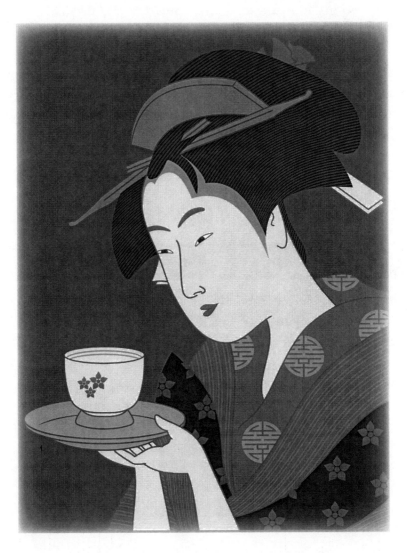

*"Remember the tea kettle – its always up to its neck
in hot water, yet it still sings!"*
-Author Unknown

Gong Fu Cha
Tea with Great Skill

According to a study that appeared in the Daily Telegraph in June 2011, the British drink 165 million cups of tea per day. That's 60.2 billion cups a year! The study also revealed that the average Briton makes his or her first cup of tea at the age of seven and a half years.

Tea Bags or Loose Tea?

For the most part, people use teabags for their practicality and ease, and it was Thomas Sullivan, a New York merchant, who in 1904 decided to start selling his teas in small handmade silk bags. His clients soon discovered they could keep their tea in the bag and just add hot water to it for the infusion.

However, today's teabags contain smaller pieces of lower quality tea leaves or tea fannings/dusts. Since the bags are small, manu-facturers opt for the smaller tea leaves. If they used larger tea leaves in the bags the leaves would be prevented from fully unfurling. Tea fannings/dusts are lower quality in taste but the bags are more practical. Unfortunately, the quality of the bag's paper further pre-vents the full taste of the tea from being absorbed.

Recently, the Japanese pyramid-shaped tea bag made its debut and is manufactured from a fine silk mesh with no staples or glue extracts to distract from the taste of the tea. The bag allows the tea leaves to unfurl, providing a very tasty cup of tea.

Loose Tea

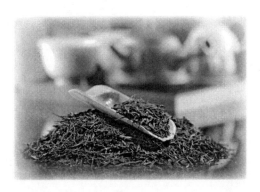

Loose tea is preferred among tea connoisseurs since it allows them to appreciate the color, fragrance and taste that larger leaves bring to a brew. The larger tea leaves take longer to unfurl and this is what gives the tea a better taste as it brews, and maximum health benefits.

The Skill of Brewing

The taste of your tea is improved when you pre-warm your teapot or mug. Throw out the water from the teapot and add your chosen tea, and fresh hot water. Let the tea steep for the right amount of time (see guidelines overleaf) and then empty the water from your cups, strain and pour your tea.

Remember, tea leaves will expand in the teapot during your first brew, so each time you refill with hot water, there will be less room for water and fewer servings.

To Boil or not to Boil your Water?

The practice in the West has always been to pour boiling water straight onto the tea, hence one of the reasons the teacup handle was invented.

This method provides a fairly decent cup of black tea with milk or sugar added; for fewer calories, just add lemon and honey. However, we would do much better to follow the traditions of the East to enjoy a more delicate and flavorsome tea if we used slightly cooler water, either using a pan to boil the water so we can see the bubbles and estimate the temperature, or let your kettle boiled water cool for three minutes before pouring over your more fragile green, white or yellow teas. Once the tea has brewed, fill each of your small teacups a quarter full so that the taste is evenly distributed, and then as you finish, fill the cup again and do this for three servings to gain the best taste from your tea.

There are now kettles available that allow precise water temperatures to be reached and maintained so that you can be gentle with your green teas. The Bonavita kettle, in particular, is highly recommended.

Water Temperatures

For Black Tea - boiling means the water has *just* reached a slow boil with big bubbles. The Chinese call this "Fish-Eye Water." The water should reach 180-190 F/ 82-92 C.

For Green tea – boil the water until small streams of tiny bubbles start to rise from the bottom of the pan or kettle. The Chinese call this "Crab-Eye Water." The water should reach 160-170 F/ 71 C – 82 C.

For *Oolong* Tea - the correct temperature for the water should reach 175 F/ 79 C.

Brewing Times:

The longer you brew a tea, the more caffeine and tannins will be released, making the tea bitter and more robust in flavor. The steeping times below are approximate and you can adjust them according to your taste. Allow 1-1½ tsps of loose tea per 8 fl oz of water.

- **Black tea** - black is the most robust of the tea varieties and can be brewed in truly boiling water, usually steeped for three to seven minutes. If you prefer your tea stronger, use more than one tea bag, and keep to the same steeping time.
- *Oolong* **tea** – *oolong* tea falls between green and black. Traditionally *oolong* should be steeped longer than black tea, for around five to eight minutes. However, those sensitive to caffeine should limit brewing time to three minutes.
- **Green tea** – be gentle with your green teas to get the most healing benefits from them. They should only be steeped for two to three minutes.
- **White tea** – a delicate tea to be handled with the greatest respect. Steep for at least four to six minutes to truly bring out its delicate flavor.
- *Pu'erh* **tea** (leaf or cake/brick) – this is a fermented tea and is deep reddish brown in color. It is prepared in the same way as black tea with boiling water, and traditionally left to steep for only 30 seconds. However, in the West we can often steep the tea for up to eight minutes for a stronger, more robust taste.

Tea Storage

When purchasing loose tea, ensure you have enough to last you for three to four weeks, and store it in small tin, or an airtight container. Store the canisters in a cool, dark and dry place; avoid storing the tea over the stove, in the freezer or refrigerator since light and moisture create enzymes in the tea that destroy the leaves.

> *"We had a kettle; we let it leak:*
> *Our not repairing made it worse.*
> *We haven't had any tea for a week ...*
> *The bottom is out of the universe."*
> *- Rudyard Kipling*

Herbal Teas
From Nature's Medicine Cabinet

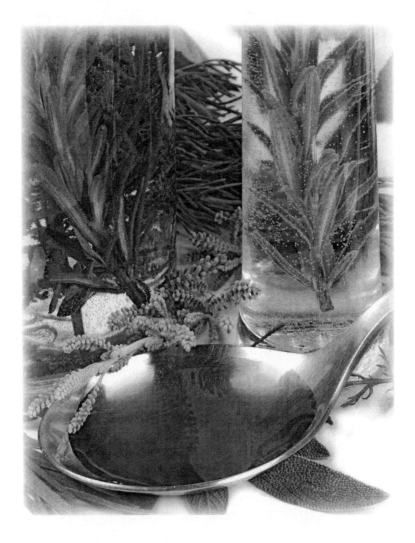

"The doctor of the future will give no medicine,
but will interest his patients in the care of the human frame,
in diet, and in the cause and prevention of disease."
-Thomas Edison

Herbal Teas

Herbal teas are a combination of fresh or dried herbs, spices, dried fruits and natural flavors. They are caffeine-free because they don't contain tea leaves. A cup of herbal tea can be warming; have therapeutic effects; be relaxing or serve as a pick-me up during a busy schedule.

Herbal teas, or tisanes as they are also known, date back to the ancient civilizations of Egypt, China, Greece and Italy where they were consumed for their medicinal, nutritional, aromatic, and religious properties.

During these times, it was quite common for monasteries, nobility and the wealthy to have their own walled herb gardens within their estate where the servants would pick herbs daily for cooking, medicines, teas, poultices, fragrances and tinctures. Indeed, in homes and estates of the wealthy, the so-called Still Room was allocated for the preparation of fresh or dried plant material.

Long before black tea ever reached European shores, the herbal tea/tisane was the drink of choice.

The medicinal uses of herbal teas are extensive and for time im-memorial, they have been used to treat every illness or disease known to mankind around the world.

For the most part, herbal teas can be consumed as a preventa-tive measure against the flu, for example, or to build immunity. Others may focus on detoxing the body, improving digestion or as a sleep-aid.

Depending on the health issue, herbs and spices are chosen for their therapeutic values. Just like tea leaves, herbs also possess phy-tochemicals that will also benefit our health and well-being.

Herbal teas, tisanes, infusions or tinctures all come under the um-brella of plant medicine, phytomedicine or herbalism, involving the preparation of organic plant materials to support health issues.

Please note it is always wise to consult with a health care practitioner before drinking herbal teas if you have a medical condition or are taking drugs. We are all unique in our chemical and emotional make-up; some teas may work for you while others may not. If you are pregnant, check the herbal ingredients listed in the tea. Sometimes a ginger tea will also have other spices or herbs that may not be appropriate for use during pregnancy.

Creating a Herbal Tea

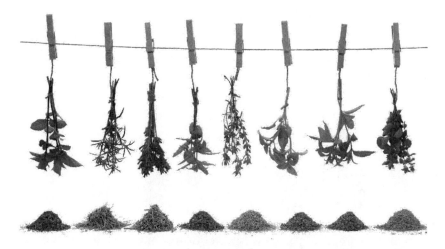

A cornucopia of delight for the senses and taste buds.

There are many herbal teas on the market from which to choose. Ideally, the single note blends like rosemary, peppermint, chamomile, ginger and lavender are the easiest to start with since they are specific to a health need, and have no other herbs or spices blended with them.

Manufacturers have also created blends of herbs, fruits and roots to promote different states of well being, and the function of the tea will be shown on the box or tea bag. These blends are delicious, combining rose petals, orange peel, lemon verbena, ginger and lavender with essential oils to add to the aroma of the tea.

When purchasing your herbal teas, check the ingredients to make sure the dried fruits and spices are natural, and not artificial.

Which Herbs?

Fresh or dried herbs will bring the vitality and nutrients from the plant to your body. However, you will gain a greater proportion of nutrients and vitamins from your herbs if you pick them fresh. Dried herbs lose their potency during the drying process. Doing your research is important in order to determine which herb could be right for you. The web provides a wealth of information; one of my favorite websites is www.plant-medicine.com.

Always Listen to Your Body!

Learn to listen to your body's wisdom. If you feel good after drinking your tea, that is a positive sign. If you feel nauseous or notice a headache coming on, avoid that particular tea. Also avoid drinking the same herbal concoction continuously; give yourself breaks as sometimes we can have too much of a good thing!

Dried Herbs

You can easily make your own customized loose herbal tea blend from the many online wholesalers of herbs and spices from around the world. A list of suppliers is at the back of the book.

Check with your supplier on the quality and freshness of their herbs, and whether they are organic. Loose herbal teas are a better buy since the warm water can circulate freely among the herbs and spices, releasing the goodness of the herbs. A herbal tea bag is more limited as the paper filters the water and less nutrients escape into your cup.

Once your tea supply has arrived, and before making yourself a cup, follow the Chinese method of washing the required amount of tea by placing it in a teapot; adding a small amount of hot water to cover the tea; swirling the water around, and then straining the water. This way you remove the dust and any other unwanted visitors in the tea before drinking it.

When you are ready to make your tea, add boiled warm water to the tea. Remember, if it is too hot, the heat will destroy some of the nutrients in the herbs.

Picking Herbs Fresh from the Garden – for quiet contemplation

To truly step into the ritual of tea, what could be better than handpicking your own herbs from the garden for a tranquil and relaxing way to begin your tea ceremony.

Pick your herbs in the morning before the midday sun evaporates the energy, vital oils and nutrients in their leaves.. A good handful of either spearmint, peppermint, lavender, lemon verbena or lemon grass washed and then steeped for about three to eight minutes in hot water is all you need for a refreshing herbal cup of tea.

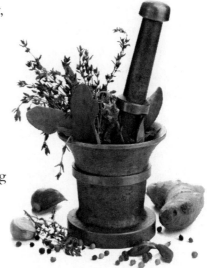

The art of preparing herbal tea in this way gives you the chance to connect with nature, relax and let go of worries. The tea's aroma and warmth can only calm and help you focus on your well-being.

Drying Herbs For Tea

Drying herbs means losing some of the potency of the plant but it allows for year-round use. The herbs can be used in cooking as well.

Pick your herbs in the morning for the highest quality, and then choose one of the following options for drying:

- **Air Drying** - this is the easiest method and is suitable for sage, thyme, dill, bay leaves, oregano, rosemary and marjoram as these herbs have low moisture content and dry quickly without going moldy.

After picking and washing your herbs, bunch them together and tie them either with an elastic band or string around the stems. Place a brown paper bag over their heads and tie this with another piece of string, not too tightly. Find a dark, dry cupboard and hang them upside down for a few weeks or until dry and crumbly. Once they have dried, you can crumble them and keep them in an airtight container for your teas or for cooking. The brown paper bag will catch any dry leaves that fall off.

- **Oven Drying** - for herbs with a higher moisture content such as basil, tarragon, lemon balm and mint, spread the herbs out on a baking tray.

Heat the oven for 20 minutes at the lowest setting and then turn it off. Put your herbs on a baking tray and into the oven for a couple of hours.

- **Freezing** - not so ideal for tea, but great for cooking. Place a teaspoon of fresh leaves in each ice cube container, cover with a ziplock bag, squeezing out the air, and freeze. This way, once frozen, you have ready- made measurements of herbs you can just pop out of the ice tray and into your cooking.

Herbal Tea Storage

Herbal teas can degrade quickly when exposed to air, light, humidity, and heat. Choose an attractive china or porcelain air-tight container to store your dried herbal teas.

Brewing Herbal Teas

In the herbal tea world, there are two methods for brewing teas.

- *Infusions – are teas made from flowers, leaves and light plant materials.*
- *Decoctions – are brewed from the bark, root, twigs, berries and seeds.*
- To make a tea infusion - put one to two tablespoons of herbal tea into a teapot. Add 6 - 8 fl oz of slightly cooled boiled water and allow to brew for up to three to five minutes. For a greater medicinal effect, brew for 15 - 30 minutes. Will keep for 24 hours when refrigerated.
- To make a tea decoction - decoctions have longer steeping times for heavier plant materials. Put one to three table-spoons of cut herb, seed, root, bark, into a pot with 16 - 32 fl oz of water and allow to sit in cool water for at least five to ten minutes. Bring the water to a slow boil then turn down to a simmer for 10-30 minutes. The time depends on the strength of tea you enjoy. Strain and drink. Will keep for approximately 72 hours when refrigerated.

Choosing Herbs and Fruits for Your Teas

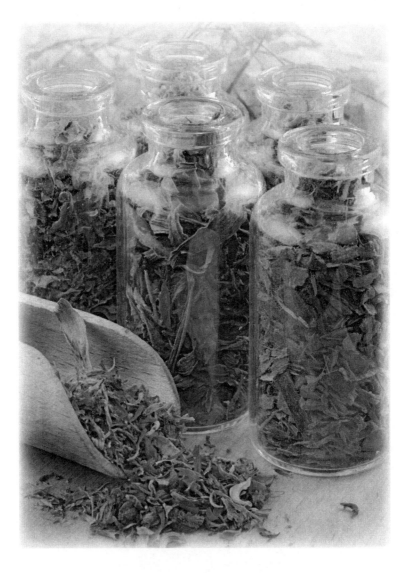

"Let thy food be thy medicine and thy medicine be thy food."
-Hippocrates (460-377 B.C.)

German Chamomile – a small gentle flower with the power to calm

Chamomile is a pretty daisy-like flower that calms the nervous system and helps you sleep. There is also a Roman/English chamomile that has a bitter taste. In aromatherapy, we use German chamomile for soothing skin disorders. It contains chamazulene, which makes the oil blue; is effective for soothing skin disorders, and is also anti–inflammatory.

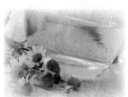

Matricaria recutita

Tea: You can benefit from the sedative flavonoids, chrysin and apigenin found in chamomile by simply adding a cup of hot water to one cup of dried or fresh flowers. Drinking a cup before bedtime will help you relax and sleep.

The Benefits: Chamomile has anti–inflammatory properties and can work in aromatherapy as a topical skin-calming agent. It has naturally occurring chemicals within it to help block pain receptors. Chamomile helps to calm nervous digestion and sooth tension.

Allergic Reactions: Adverse reactions to chamomile can occur if you are allergic to the ragweed family. Other herbs you may also be allergic to in the Asteracea family include: Arnica, Dandelion, Echinacea, Feverfew and Milk Thistle.

Cranberry Fruit – a berry good bladder healer

Native to North America, cranberries grow on long-running vines in sandy bogs. It was the Native American Indians who used cranberries for their medicinal benefits and for dying their clothes. It is believed that the pilgrims served cranberries at the first Thanksgiving, thus beginning the time-held tradition.

Dutch and German settlers first called this berry "crane-berry" as the flowers on the vine resembled the bill of a crane. Cranberries are wet-harvested by flooding the bog with a few inches of water. "Egg-beaters" then go into the bog and loosen the berries from the vines. The berries float to the surface of the water, which are scooped up. The fresh berries you see in the stores are dry harvested by a machine to keep them whole and tender.

Tea: You can benefit from cranberry tea if you have a urinary tract infection by simply boiling two cups of cranberries with two cups of water in a pan for 5-10 minutes. Then when the cranberries are soft, you can mash and strain them to separate the juice from the pulp. If the concentrate tastes too strong, add more water, and sweeten with honey. Add lemon to make the tea really cleansing. For a quicker and simpler method, add two tablespoons of unsweetened cranberry juice to your green tea for a super healthy antioxidant-packed drink.

The Benefits: Cranberries contain proanthocyanidins (PACs) that can prevent the adhesion of certain bacteria, including *E. coli*, associated with urinary tract infections. Cranberry's anti-adhesion properties may inhibit the bacteria associated with gum disease and stomach ulcers. Cranberries contain significant amounts of antioxidants and phytonutrients that may help protect against heart disease and cancer.

Dandelion - a mighty weed for the liver

This powerful little weed was recommended by Arab physicians in the eleventh century to clear toxicity from the body. All parts of this plant are used for their healing benefits. The leaves are juiced, eaten raw or dried and have a diuretic effect on the body.

Dandelion leaves have high levels of potassium and will replenish the body with this mineral rather than deplete it as conventional diuretics can do. The leaves also have an effect on the gallbladder, helping to dissolve or prevent gallstones. Seek the advice of a professional herbalist if you choose to use dandelion in this way. The root , fresh or dried, has a significant cleansing action on the liver.

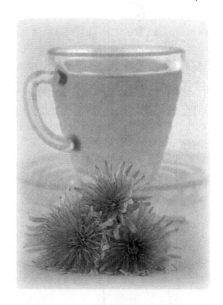

Taraxacum officinale

Tea: You can benefit from a cup of dandelion tea by picking it fresh, ideally from your own garden. Wash and put a handful in a tea pot, cover with cup of freshly boiled water, and allow the tea to steep for at least 10 minutes before straining into your warmed cup. Drink two cups a day for about six weeks.

The Benefits: Dandelion contains vitamins A, B-complex, C, E, biotin, calcium, choline, inositol, iron, linolenic acid, magnesium, niacin, PABA, phosphorus, potassium, zinc and sulfur. The tea may increase the free flow of urine; aid digestion; improve the function of the pancreas; and may help against cirrhosis of the liver, hepatitis, and hypoglycemia.

The inulin in the root can encourage the growth of beneficial intestinal bacteria and may halt tumor development.

Allergic Reactions: Avoid dandelion if you are allergic to the ragweed family of plants.

Echinacea – supports the emperor of your castle – your immune system

Native to North America, echinacea has been used for centuries by Native American Indians for its antiseptic qualities and for toothaches.

Today we use it to strengthen the body's immune system so we can prevent viral and bacterial infections. It is the root, dried or fresh, that helps the immune system. The flower from the plant can be used for fighting infections.

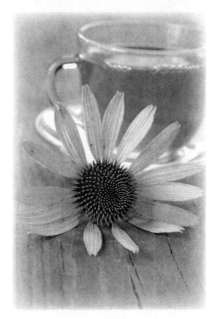

Echinacea angustifolia & E purpurea

Tea: You can benefit from the tea by using freeze dried or powdered Echinacea. Take one cup of freshly boiled water to one teaspoon of tea; allow it to steep for five minutes before straining it into your cup. If you can use the fresh root, then follow the decoction brewing instructions. You can drink the tea daily as a preventative measure, or if there are viral infections at work or at home, or you succumb to the flu, drink two cups daily for no longer than six to eight weeks. See below for when to avoid Echinacea.

The Benefits: Echinacea contains alkamides that are antibacterial and antifungal; caffeic acid esters and polysaccharides, which inhibit viruses from taking over cells in the body. Also known to to reduce inflammation, the herb is antibiotic and can help to detox, heal wounds and fight the effects of M.E. (myalgic encephalomyelitis). It is also effective as a gargle for throat infections and for treating allergies.

Allergic Reactions: If you are allergic to the ragweed family, avoid using echinacea. Also if you notice itchy eyes, vomiting, dizziness or shortness of breath, stop taking it.

Also avoid echinacea if you have chronic inflammatory diseases or autoimmune diseases: Diabetes, Type 1, Crohn's disease, Thyroid disease, Lupus, Myasthenia gravis, MS, Ankylosing Spondilitis and Rheumatoid Arthritis.

Echinacea enhances the growth and activation of immune cells. However, it also stimulates the growth of blood vessels that feed tumors, so in the case of advanced cancers and AIDS, it is best avoided. (Herbs DeMystified, Holly Phaneuf, PhD.)

Garlic - your aromatic heart doctor

This may come as a surprise but garlic is from the same family as the lily that grows in your garden. It is the sulfur content in garlic that creates the pungent odor, and once the garlic has been chopped, it is the sulfurous molecules that sting your eyes and make them water.

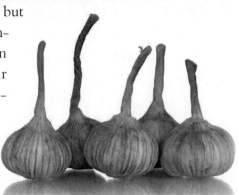

Allium sativum

The molecules are so strong that even rubbing a clove of garlic on your feet will bring the taste of garlic to your breath within minutes if you use enough of it!

Garlic may lower blood pressure by opening up blood vessels and will also work to clear blockages in the sinuses by making your nose run. Garlic can increase good cholesterol, (HDL) and can also reduce bad cholesterol. Garlic's sulfur molecules are excellent at eating up free radicals, protecting cells from damaging toxins that cause our healthy cells to mutate into cancer cells.

Tea: You can benefit from the tea by drinking it to ward off symptoms of colds and respiratory infections, or just as a daily health drink. Chop three large garlic cloves and let them infuse in two cups of boiling water for three minutes or more, depending on your preference. Strain the liquid into a cup, and add half a lemon and honey to taste. If you are really daring, you can also eat the boiled cloves … but you may want to avoid socializing.

The Benefits: Traditionally, garlic has always been valued for its curative powers. Even before antibiotics, garlic was being used to treat tuberculosis, typhoid and to dress wounds during World War I. Today, garlic helps chest infections, colds, flu, ear infections, digestive infections, removes parasites, thins the blood, reduces blood sugar levels and prevents clotting. It can be taken alongside antibiotics.

Allergic Reactions: Avoid garlic if you are taking blood-thinning medications as garlic thins the blood, and ask your doctor if you should avoid it at least one week before surgery in order to minimize excessive bleeding.

Ginger – a friend to warm and help you digest

Used for many centuries, ginger is renowned for its motion sickness, digestive, and circulatory benefits. In Chinese medicine, the herb is dried and used for those with "internal cold" symptoms including cold hands, weak pulse, and a pale complexion. The fresh herb is used for fever, headaches, and aching muscles.

Ginger contains gingerol, a constituent which gives it a hot taste and stimu-

Zingiber officinale

lates blood flow, thus improving circulation in the hands and feet. A powerful antiseptic, ginger has been used to treat dysentery and relieve postoperative nausea. For pregnant women, ginger can reduce morning sickness.

Tea: You can benefit from ginger tea by drinking one cup a day for nausea. If you have motion sickness, take some tea in the car or drink it an hour before travelling. Dried ginger or candied ginger root may also help on the journey. To make a decoction of ginger, you need to grate a ½ oz of ginger root and put it into a pan with two cups of water and simmer for at least 10 minutes. Strain and serve with honey and lemon for a well-known effective cold remedy. Without the honey and lemon, it is also an effective tea for indigestion and stomach cramps, or abdominal bloating.

The Benefits: Ginger tea may improve dizziness, colic, and may even be beneficial for intestinal infections. Ginger can improve joint movement and reduce arthritis pain.

Allergic Reactions: Ginger may reduce the blood's ability to clot (ginger has constituents that resemble aspirin). It is advisable to check with your healthcare provider, particularly if you are taking aspirin, before drinking ginger tea.

Hibiscus – to open your heart and balance your blood pressure

Hibiscus tea is made from the sepals of the hibiscus flower and its tart cranberry-like flavor is enjoyed by a diversity of cultures around the world, including Jamaica, Mexico, Central and South America, and the Caribbean where they add ginger and sugar to it, and sometimes rum! In the Sudan and Upper Egypt, hibiscus tea is prized and is used to toast married couples at wedding celebrations.

Ancient Egyptians believed that hibiscus could bring about feelings of lust in women, so they were forbidden to wear the flower.

However, if a man were to wear a hibiscus flower behind his left ear, it meant he was looking for a wife; and if he wore it behind the right ear, it meant he was married!

Tea: You can benefit from the antioxidants (high levels of Vitamin C) and the phytosterols which lower cholesterol, by either purchasing the loose dried flowers (available at Mexican markets (called "Flor de Jamaica"), or order online. See suppliers list.

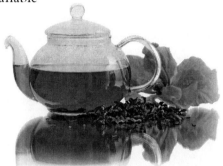

To make dried hibiscus tea, add one teaspoon of the dried flowers to one cup of hot water, allowing it to

Hibiscus sabdariffa

steep for three to five minutes, depending on your taste. Once you have strained the tea, add half a cinnamon stick, some lime juice, and a little sugar to add some zing to this very pretty tea.

You can make your own fresh hibiscus tea by picking a single flower that includes the calyx (this is the red fleshy cup that holds the flower). After washing the calyx, place it in your teapot, and fill with one cup of boiling water. Allow the flower to steep for 10 minutes before straining the tea into your cup.

The Benefits: Long used for high-blood pressure, hibiscus tea has received scientific attention for its ability to treat mild hypertension.

A study published in the February 2010 issue of the *Journal of Nutrition* found that participants, aged 30 to 70 who consumed three 240 milliliter servings of brewed hibiscus tea per day for six weeks, showed lower blood pressure readings at the end of the ex-periment. Hibiscus tea reduced both systolic pressure -- the upper number of the blood pressure ratio, which represents the pressure in the blood vessels when the heart contracts -- and diastolic -- the lower number, which represents the pressure in the blood vessels during relaxation of the heart.

The researchers concluded that hibiscus tea effectively lowers blood pressure with doses that can easily be incorporated into the average person's diet.

The University of Maryland Medical Center also supports drink-ing hibiscus tea to lower blood pressure and recommends brewing two tablespoons of dried hibiscus flower per cup of water.

Fibromyalgia: Malic acid, which gives hibiscus tea its sour taste, has been studied as a possible treatment for fibromyalgia symp-toms. A 1995 study published in the *Journal of Rheumatology* found that a malic acid supplement safely reduced pain and tenderness in those with fibromyalgia.

Kidneys: Hibiscus tea also helps the kidneys, according to a study cited in the *Journal of Ethnopharmacology* in 2008, which concluded that the tea improved the kidney's ability to filter out waste prod-ucts that could potentially form kidney stones. Participants drank one cup of tea twice a day for 15 days. Those who had previously experienced kidney stones showed elevated waste products in their urine. When they stopped drinking the tea, the level of waste products declined.

Allergic Reactions: Avoid hibiscus if you are allergic to hibiscus or other plants in the malvaceae family (okra, cotton, cacao) and if you have low blood pressure or are taking blood pressure medication (consult your doctor first). Hibiscus tea may have estrogenic actions, and those on hormone re-placement therapy or on birth control pills should be cautious. In addition, hibiscus tea may interfere with anti-inflammatory drugs such as acetamino-phen. Your doctor may recommend a two -hour waiting period before drink-ing hibiscus tea, after taking your anti-inflammatory medication.

Lavender – to comfort and relax

With over 2,500 years of documented use, the evocative and ar-omatic lavender has been widely used for washing, perfuming, cooking, and to calm the mind. It is believed that lavender was first domesticated in Arabia and found its way to the Mediterranean with Greek traders about 600 B.C.

Surprising to some, lavender belongs to the mint family, and like other varieties of this family, is helpful in calming digestive issues. Lavender also has a soothing effect on the nervous system and in my work, I have noted its balancing and calming effect on PTSD (Post Traumatic Stress Disorder) and autism, combined with Reiki.

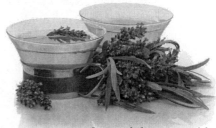

The primary compound in lavender is called linalool, one of the molecules that

Lavandula angustifolia

gives lavender its distinctive calming properties. Linalool is known to calm the brain. More is given later in the book about lavender essential oil, along with some remedies.

Tea: You can make a tea from dried lavender flowers and leaves. Large quantities of volatile essential oil are contained in the

flowering buds, therefore it is safer to dry the flowers first by hanging bunches of lavender upside down with their florets in a dark
cupboard for about three to four weeks. Tie a brown paper bag
over it so that the dried florets collect inside it. When they are
dried, you can shred the flowers and leaves straight into the bag
without losing your stash!

For restlessness, fatigue, nervousness, insomnia, indigestion and
gas, take one or two teaspoons of the dried flowers and leaves and
steep in one cup of boiling water for 10 minutes or longer. Strain
the tea and drink two to three cups daily with one teaspoon of
honey before retiring at night.

You can also fill small muslin bags with the dried lavender to keep
moths out of your closet, and under your pillow.

The Benefits: Traditional and current uses for lavender include
its ability to reduce anxiety, headaches, migraines, and in cases of
asthma attributed to nervousness, it may reduce attacks and ease
their severity. Lavender is also known for its ability to relieve muscle tension.

*Allergic Reactions: Avoid lavender if you suffer from acute low blood pres-
sure. Avoid using lavender in high dosages as it may cause an allergic
reaction.*

Lemon Balm - improves memory, uplifts moods, chases cold sores away

From the mint family, lemon balm has a delicious refreshingly
lemony fragrance with a minty touch that immediately uplifts
your mood and chases away the clouds.

The herb attracts many bees to its tiny white flowers hence its Greek name *Melissa,* which means bee. You can harvest most of the leaves from the plant and yet in a few weeks it will thrive once again, ready to help us if we feel a cold or flu coming on.

Used for centuries, lemon balm has been known to relieve cold sores, owing to its polyphenols and tannins that may account for many of the herb's antiviral effects. These help to re-

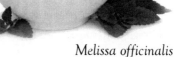

Melissa officinalis

duce the healing time of cold sores and reduce further outbreaks.

The herb also has an effect on overactive thyroids and has been indicated to possibly slow down the thyroid by altering the TSH structure (Thyroid Stimulating Hormone), thereby helping to reduce its production.

Tea: Steep one tablespoon of fresh herbs or one to two teaspoons of dried herbs in one cup of boiling water and allow to brew for three minutes. Strain the tea and drink one to three cups daily. You can also use the tea for cold sores by applying the tea - once it has cooled - to the sore with a cotton tip until it has dried up.

The Benefits: Lemon Balm can improve cognitive performance and mood. Research has shown that using the herb might be an additional therapy for Alzheimer's. A study published in the October 2003 *Neuropsychopharmacology* issue revealed that in a randomized, double-blind, placebo-controlled trial involving 20 healthy participants, the researchers found that using 1,600 mg of lemon balm improved memory performance, and had a calming effect.

According to the University of Maryland Medical Center, lemon balm has been tested also on individuals diagnosed with mild to moderate Alzheimer's disease, and positive findings were recorded in managing cognitive function when taken in daily doses.

Lemon balm is a relaxing tonic and is useful when over-anxiety can create digestive issues. The herb may also calm a racing heart when stress is involved.

It is not recommended to self-treat either Alzheimer's or Graves Disease with lemon balm tea. However, drinking the tea sporadically may not be problematic. Consult your health care practitioner.

Marshmallow – soothes away intestinal troubles, coughs and sore throats

As it name indicates, marshmallow grows in marshes. The marshmallow puff candy that we toast around the fire was once made from the roots of a plant from the mallow family.

Reportedly used as far back as 372-286 B.C. by the Greeks, the marshmallow root was steeped in sweet wine and used for coughs.

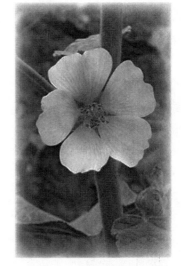

Owing to its slimy or mucilage properties, once marshmallow powder is mixed with water, it turns into a spongy slime that helps to protect mucus linings within the body. For example, in the case of excess stomach

Althea officinalis

acid or ulcers, marshmallow will form a fine layer on the surface of the stomach, protecting it from irritants and allowing the body to heal the affected area. It could be compared to putting a band aid on a cut. This shields the wound from invading bacteria and germs, and gives it a chance to heal.

Tea: You can benefit from the mucilage and mild laxative properties of marshmallow by infusing a teaspoon of dried marshmallow leaves in one cup of cooled boiled water. Allow the infusion to stand overnight, strain the liquid into a saucepan and heat very gently until it is just warm. Overheating can destroy the mucilaginous properties. Drink two to three cups per day.

The Benefits: Colitis, Diverticulitis, and Irritable Bowel Syndrome are soothed by drinking marshmallow tea. For dry coughs, asthma, bronchial congestion and sore throats, the tea will help soothe, but not cure any infections.

Peppermint – breathe ... hear your body sigh with relief

Dried peppermint leaves were found in Egyptian pyramids dating back to approximately 1,000 B.C. However, peppermint only made its debut in Europe in the eighteenth century where it was widely used for the treatment of gas, bloating and colic.

Its uses are extensive, making it a very versatile herb, and of course it is the prime ingredient in Moroccan tea. See page 24 for recipe details.

Peppermint contains high levels of menthol, menthone, and methyl acetate, which are known to help relax involuntary muscles such as those lining our digestive tracts. Peppermint is useful in treating certain types of indigestion, including IBS with chronic diarrhea, constipation, gas and bloating.

For constipation, you might want to drink peppermint tea in moderation. The tea is effective in cases of constipation caused by erratic bowel muscle movement due to stress or illness. However, if constipation is caused by a sluggish digestive system where the muscles are already relaxed, then peppermint tea could make it worse.

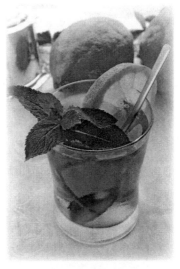

Mentha piperita

Tea: You can benefit from peppermint tea by taking one full teaspoon of dried herbs or a tablespoon of fresh leaves with one cup of boiling water. Steep for 10 minutes before straining the leaves. Drink the tea three to four times a day.

The Benefits: Drink the tea if you suffer from nausea, headaches, indigestion or gas. For sinus congestion and breathing problems, peppermint tea may open the sinus passages with its stimulating properties. The menthol in peppermint can open passages in the lungs by relaxing the involuntary muscles around the bronchioles.

Allergic Reactions: If you take cholesterol-lowering drugs or blood pressure medications, peppermint tea may interfere with them. Check with your health care practitioner before drinking the tea. Peppermint oil in high dosages may increase blood pressure.

Pomegranate – a red ruby of health

The pomegranate's history dates back to biblical times. Its name is derived from the French *pomme granate* or "seeded apple." Believed to have originated in Iran, the pomegranate is an ancient fruit, and is even thought to be the real forbidden fruit cited in the Bible's Garden of Eden. The ancients revered it as the symbol of life after death, and also for fertility.

Today, research has shown that when taken daily as a juice or tea, the antioxidant-rich pomegranate can slow the buildup of cholesterol in the arteries. Pomegranate is also known to reduce bad cholesterol (LDL) and help lower blood pressure.

Punica granatum

The polyphenols, tannins and anthocyanins in the pomegranate make it very good for us as we need these chemicals to fight off toxins.

Pomegranate can help with skin care issues including age spots, dry skin, pigmentation and acne break-outs. It also has compounds that protect the skin against free radical damage, helping to prevent skin cancer and relieving sunburn. Pomegranate oil inhibits the growth of skin tumors, according to the Probelte Bio Laboratory. The fruit juice and extract also slow down the wear and tear of DNA, a major contributing factor to aging.

Tea: You can benefit from the tea by either juicing pomegranate seeds, (some stores sell them already separated from the fruit), and adding your freshly squeezed juice to black or green tea. Or you can purchase fresh pomegranate juice and add a teaspoon at a time to your cup of tea, adjusting the taste as you go. Drink two cups daily.

Drinking iced pomegranate tea in the hot summer months makes for an exceptionally refreshing and healthy drink.

The Benefits: In addition to the above, research reported in the *Journal of Ethnopharmacology*, pomegranate has been said to be helpful for women dealing with menopause-related depression. Pomegranates contain thiamine, niacin, vitamin C, calcium, and phosphorus, all of which provide us with a great immune support system against colds and the flu.

Case Western Reserve University School of Medicine proved that eating pomegranates slowed down joint conditions such as osteoarthritis.

Allergic Reactions: Pomegranate, as with grapefruit juice, can adversely interact with certain drugs. Pomegranate is less potent than grapefruit. However, if your prescriptions include such medications as an anti-hyper-tensive, a statin, an ACE inhibitor or warfarin, check with your health care provider before making pomegranate juice a regular part of your diet.

Raspberry Leaf – empowering your femininity

For centuries, women drank raspberry tea to tone their uterine muscles for the rigors of childbirth and afterwards, to help the uterus return to its normal state.

Using raspberry tea may also help regulate menstrual cycles and enhance fertility.

Raspberry leaves contain many nutrients, including citric acid, iron, potassium, calcium and vitamins A, B, C and E. The herb is known to help ease uterine pain and menstrual cramps, and it may even prevent miscarriage. The leaves contain fragrine, an alkaloid, which can nourish and tone the uterine muscles and create more effective con-

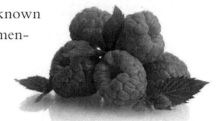

Rubus idaeus

tractions during labor and birth, and improve recovery after labor.

Tea: You can benefit from the tea by pouring a cup of boiling water over an ounce of dried raspberry leaves and brew for up to 30 minutes. Strain the tea, and add honey and lemon. Drink one to two cups daily. Having it iced also makes for a refreshing thirst quencher in the summer.

The Benefits: Many women claim that drinking red raspberry leaf tea has helped them to give birth easily, especially if combined with a healthy diet and regular exercise. According to research by the University of Maryland Medical Center, raspberry leaf tea has proven to be effective against diarrhea as it has a drying effect on the mucous membranes of the intestines, encouraging regular bowel movements.

Despite being suggested for morning sickness, there is still some controversy about whether the tea should be used throughout pregnancy. Many health care providers and the American Pregnancy Association therefore recommend drinking red raspberry leaf tea only from the second trimester.

Rooibos Tea – for your immune system and for relieving stress

Rooibos is a herbal, caffeine-free tea that was used as a substitute for real tea during World War II when tea supplies from Asia were difficult to secure.

The South African *rooibos* or red bush leaves are fermented in the same way as tea leaves. The process gives the leaves a reddish brown color and enhances the flavor. The leaves contain high levels of anti-oxidants, are caffeine-free and have very low tannin levels compared to oxidized black tea leaves.

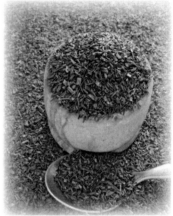

It was in 1772 that the Swedish bot-anist Carl Thunberg noted that the local people in the Cederberg re-gion in South Africa were making tea from a plant related to the red bush. The needle-like leaves were

Aspalathus linearis

picked from the wild *rooibos* plants and then rolled and put into hessian bags and brought down the mountain. They were then bruised and chopped and left to dry in the sun.

Since black tea was expensive, the Dutch settlers in South Africa decided to make *rooibos* their own tea. It was in 1904 when Benjamin Ginsberg, a Russian, perfected the curing of *rooibos* tea by copying the Chinese method of fermenting tea. In the case of *rooibos* tea, they covered it in wet, hessian sacking to ferment instead of the bamboo baskets that were used to make the fine *keemun* tea in China.

Tea: You can benefit from the tea by pouring a cup of boiling water over one teaspoon of dried *rooibos* leaves and brew for up to three minutes. Strain the tea and add honey, lemon, or a cinnamon stick. Drink one to two cups daily.

The Benefits: Research undertaken in Japan showed that *rooibos* can boost the immune system because it has proven to be antimutagenic, anticarcinogenic, anti-inflammatory and antiviral. Quercetin is the primary super-antioxidant in the tea known to benefit the heart, reduce certain types of cancer, and ease inflammation in the body.

The tea's nothofagin (antioxidant) properties have a calming effect on the body as they suppress the output of adrenal hormones. Drinking the tea daily can help relieve tension, irritation, insomnia, and even high blood pressure.

Rooibos also contains aspalathin, an antioxidant that regulates blood sugar; making it effective in managing Diabetes, Type 2.

Rooibos also has its "green tea" version where the leaves are unoxidised and provide a good source of iron, potassium, zinc, sodium, and manganese.

To keep your skin clear and radiant, *rooibos* may be beneficial when the cooled tea is applied to skin problems, including sunburn, eczema, and rashes since the tea contains powerful antioxidants. *Rooibos,* as with green and white tea, can also be used to slow down the process of aging.

Rose Damask – for love of self and love of others

This absolutely beautiful rose has been long revered for its perfume and is harvested for its oil known as "rose otto," "rose absolute," or "rose attar." The largest producing areas are Kazanlak in Bulgaria, and Turkey. A Turkish judge is reported to have brought the rose to Bulgaria in the 1500s and began to cultivate the rose in his garden. Kazanlak is now called the "Valley of the Roses." Bulgarian rose otto and Bulgarian rose oil are now commercially grown there.

In Turkey, rose oil is known as an *attar*.

Extracting the oil from thousands of tons of petals is an expensive process, hence the high price ticket on Turkish rose oil.

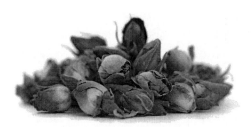

Rosa damascena

However, India is now producing a less expensive rose oil, possibly due to lower labor costs.

The flower originates from the Middle East were it was acclaimed by the Arabs for its beauty and representation of love. It is said to have been brought to England by crusader Robert de Brie around 1254 from the city of Damascus, Syria.

Damask roses are accepted as being the safest for ingestion, and in the Middle East, powdered roses and rose water are added to meats and desserts to give a sweet floral flavor and fragrance.

When using rosewater in your cooking, make sure to buy the purest form without chemicals and synthetics.

Tea: Make a rose tea by putting a teaspoon of dried rose buds into your teapot and adding a cup of boiling water. Allow the tea to steep for five minutes before straining it into your cup. You may also add rosehips from the rose bush for added flavor. Rosehips and rose petals are known to have high levels of Vitamin C. However, the petals can lose up to ninety percent of their antioxidants in the drying process therefore the young tiny buds are favored for their optimum flavor and restorative properties.

To increase the level of antioxidants in the tea, mix the rose buds with loose green tea.

The Benefits: Although no direct claims have been made, drinkers of the tea report a feeling of calm and improved digestion. The tea's Vitamin C content has also been shown to strengthen the immune system and promote healthy skin.

The Tea Artisan –
Creating Your Own Tea

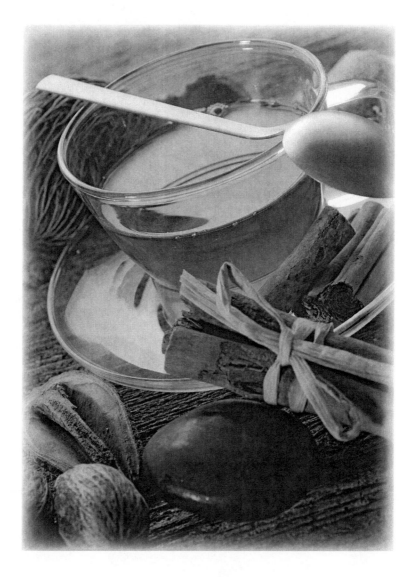

"A work of art that did not begin in emotion is not art."
-Paul Cezanne

Let your Inner Tea Chef Shine

Creating a teacup full of color, aroma
and taste ... with a little help from nature ... is a beautiful thing

For me, creating a palette of taste, fragrance, and color in one cup is pure artistry!

You can jazz your taste buds by becoming a tea chef right in your very own kitchen. Try adding a teaspoon of white, green, or black loose tea to a selection of dried orange or lemon peel slivers with dried cranberries or even blueberries. Then splash a drop of essential oil and feel your taste buds burst. with delight.

Later in the book, you will find more unique heatlth and beauty-enhancing tea recipes to create in your own kitchen.

To get you started, here are a few herbal tea blends.

Calming/Night Time Tea

Ingredients
8 fl oz boiled water
½ tsp loose dried chamomile
½ tsp loose dried lavender,
or ½ tsp of dried lemon balm
¼ tsp of honey

Preparation
1. Fill your teapot with hot water and warm it for 30 seconds. Wash your herbs.
2. Swirl the water in the pot and then discard the water.
3. Add your herbs and fill the pot with 8 fl oz of hot water and allow to brew for 3-4 minutes.
4. Add the honey to your cup then strain the tea into your cup and enjoy.

Colds and Flu/Sore Throat

Ingredients
8 fl oz water
4 slices of fresh ginger peeled
¼ tsp of lemon zest
1 slice of lemon
1 tsp of honey

Preparation
1. Peel and cut four slices of fresh ginger, grate the outer peel of the lemon and then cut a lemon slice.
2. Fill your teapot with hot water and allow to warm for 30 seconds. Swirl the water in the pot and then discard.
3. Add the ginger and grated lemon zest to the pot.
4. Fill the pot with 8 fl oz of hot water and allow to brew for 8 minutes.
5. Place the lemon slice in a mug with one tsp of honey and strain the tea into your cup.

To Warm – good for chills and stomach flu

Ingredients

8 fl oz hot water

1 tsp of *Rooibus tea*

1 pinch of ginger powder

1 pinch of cinammon

1 pinch of clove

¼ tsp of grated orange zest

¼ tsp of honey, if preferred

Preparation

1. Fill your teapot with hot water and allow to warm for 30 seconds. Swirl the water in the pot and then discard.
2. Add all ingredients to the pot and fill with 8 fl oz of hot water and allow to brew for three minutes or longer, depending on how spicy you like your tea.
3. Strain into your cup.

Digestive Ease

Ingredients
8 fl oz hot water
1 handful/tablespoon of fresh peppermint leaves
1 handful/tablespoon of fresh lemon balm leaves
¼ tsp of honey

Preparation
1. Pick your herbs, wash them.
2. Fill your teapot with hot water and allow to warm for 30 seconds.
3. Swirl the water in the pot and then discard. Add the herbs and fill the pot with 8 fl oz of hot water and allow to brew for 8 minutes.
4. Add the honey to your cup and then strain the tea onto the honey.

ᒼ ᒷ Headaches ᒼ ᒷ

Ingredients
½ tsp of loose lavender
½ tsp of loose dried peppermint
½ tsp of loose white tea leaves
¼ tsp of honey if preferred

Preparation
1. Fill your teapot with hot water and allow to warm for 30 seconds. Swirl the water in the pot and discard. Add the herbs and tea.
2. Fill the pot with 8.5 fl oz of hot water and brew for 3–5 minutes.
3. Place the honey in the cup and strain the tea into the cup.

Heart Calm – for high blood pressure

Ingredients

1 hibiscus flower or ½ tsp of dried hibiscus

¼ tsp of dried loose rose buds

¾ tsp of loose white tea

¼ tsp of honey, if preferred

Preparation

1. Pick one fresh hibiscus flower with its calyx and wash it.
2. Fill your teapot with hot water and allow to warm for 1 minute; add the fresh flower or dried hibiscus along with the loose rose buds and white tea.
3. Fill the pot with 8 fl oz of hot water and allow to brew for eight minutes.
4. Place the honey in a cup and strain the tea.

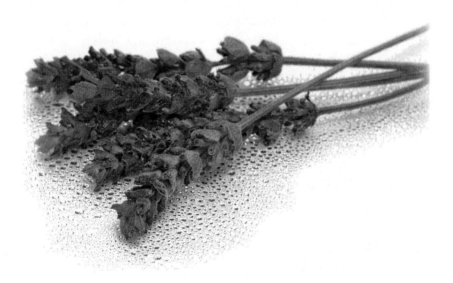

Creating Tea Blends with Essential Oils

Magic your tea into an aromatic elixir

The beauty of adding pure essential oils to your blend is the certainty that you are not adding a synthetic chemical or flavor to it, Unfortunately, not all tea manufacturers are as scrupulous.

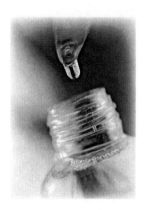

Essential oils come directly to us from nature, as do tea leaves. We are using the oils from different plant materials to add fragrance and flavor to our teas and for their health-giving properties.

I prefer to add one drop of the chosen essential oil to a dried herbal tea blend, or a traditional black, green, *oolong* or white tea. The dried tea leaves absorb the oil, and when you add the water, the heat will break down some of the oil's potency, creating a delicate aroma and taste. This way, you are not consuming the large amount of concentrated natural phytochemicals stored within the oil.

To demonstrate the potency of an essential oil, if you were to add just one drop of peppermint essential oil to a teapot filled with water, it would make at least15 - 20 cups of peppermint tea. A rule of thumb with aromatherapy is to use fewer drops of essential oil to achieve a positive result. Less is always best.

Note: Always use wildcrafted, organic, or certified therapeutic essential oils for tea. Add the oil just prior to making the tea and not ahead of time as the oil can evaporate, losing its fragrance and flavor. Never use synthetic oils or those that you would use to perfume a room.

Tea Recipes with Essential Oils

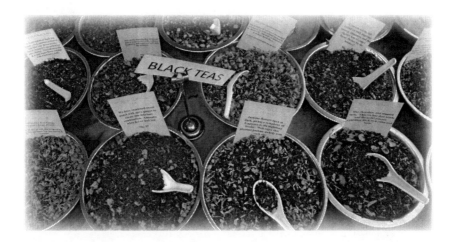

You can use, black, green, white, *oolong* or *rooibos* teas to concoct exciting blends with essential oils. Green *matcha* doesn't work so well for my palate, but have a try anyway. Your kitchen is your lab!

Always gently stir the essential oil into the tea leaves, making sure not to break them. The essential oils listed here are therapeutic grade. The brewing times shown account for the addition of essential oils that will evaporate quickly in hot water.

Oolong, White or Green Tea with Peppermint

Add a drop of peppermint essential oil to one tsp. of oolong, white or green tea. Put the blend in the teapot and then add 8 fl oz boiled water. Brew for three minutes. Strain. Delicious served warm or cold over ice with sugar and lemon.

Green or Black Tea with Sweet Orange

1. Add two drops of sweet orange essential oil to a teaspoon of green or black tea; add the blend to the teapot and then fill with 8 fl oz of hot water.
2. Allow to brew for two minutes. The orange should slightly sweeten the tea.
3. If you prefer it sweeter, add a tiny amount of honey. For added depth, include a few shreds of dried or fresh orange peel. Strain and enjoy.

Oolong, Green or White Tea with Lavender

1. Add a drop of Bulgarian lavender essential oil to a teaspoon of *oolong,* green or white tea. Stir and add the blend to the teapot.
2. Add 8 fl oz of slightly cooled boiled water and brew for three to five minutes.
3. Strain. You may need to add honey to sweeten.

⟨ ⟩ Black Tea with Bergamot ⟨ ⟩

1. Add two drops of Bergamot essential oil to one teaspoon of black tea. Add to the teapot and pour in 8 fl oz of slightly cooled boiled water.
2. Brew for two to three minutes. Congratulations, you have just made your very own Earl Grey tea!
3. Strain and add milk if required.

⟨ ⟩ Lemon Tea ⟨ ⟩

1. Add three drops of lemon essential oil to one teaspoon of any tea; pour in 8 fl oz of slightly cooled boiled water.
2. Brew for three to five minutes; for black tea two to three minutes. You can add shreds of dried or fresh lemon peel to the dried tea before brewing to amplify the citrus flavor.
3. Allow to cool, strain, and serve over ice with a twist of lemon and honey if required.

⟨ ⟩ Rooibus Tea and Ginger ⟨ ⟩

1. Add one drop of ginger to a teaspoon of *rooibus* tea, with 8 oz of boiling water.
2. Steep for three minutes, strain and drink warm.
3. To spice up the blend, combine dried or fresh orange peel with one clove and add to the dried tea before brewing.

Black or Rooibus Tea with Vanilla Essence

1. Add one drop of vanilla essential oil, or baking essence, to two teaspoons of black or *rooibos* tea; add 1 ½ cups of boiling water, and steep for two to three minutes.
2. You can also add shreds of dried orange peel to the dried tea before serving, to make this a sweet blend; strain and serve with milk. This makes a tasty tea for children.

Rose or Jasmine Fragranced Tea

I would recommend adding a drop of either rose or jasmine essential oil to a folded small square of tissue; place this in an airtight canister, and add a tablespoon of your chosen tea: green, white or black. This method will impart a delicate floral flavor and is safer than using luxury essential oils, which are often extracted using solvents. Avoid mixing absolute essential oils directly with tea. Use the method above.

Essential Oils For Your
Health and Well-being

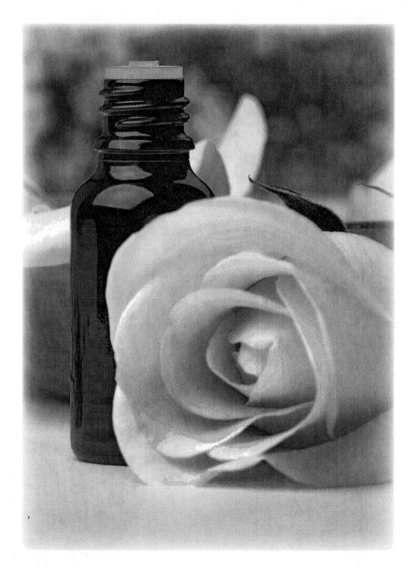

"I must have flowers, always, and always."
- Claude Monet

Using Essential Oils for Your Well-being

As you begin to explore the world of essential oils and using them in your teas, you may want to expand your knowledge of this ancient healing art. The use of essential oils is known as aroma-therapy. In aromatherapy there is an art, wisdom and science that comes with using essential oils

The art comes in blending essential oils to flavor and fragrance your teas and food; or to create aromatic elixirs and fragrances to change your mood, or perhaps ease a health issue. Their impact on your senses will, over time, help you develop an appreciation for the subtle depths of aroma and the beauty of subtlety not only in fragrances, but also in life. Once tried and tested, essential oils may even turn you against artificial fragrances for good.

The science of essential oils reaches far back to ancient times where essential oils were used for health , beauty and during ceremonies. Today, essential oils are being investigated – just as herbs are – for their health giving properties.

The natural healing compounds found in essential oils are more potent than dried herbs and therefore require only a tiny amount in your tea blends.

There are often between 70 to 300 naturally occurring compounds found in the total composition of an essential oil. These
properties give the oil a host of key therapeutic actions, making
it either: antibacterial, antifungal, antidepressant, anti-infectious,
astringent, antiseptic, anti-inflammatory, antiviral, detoxifying,
blood pressure-regulating and sedating, and sometimes a combination of all or some of these.

Their overlapping features give essential oils their holistic and heterogenetic properties, which benefit both humans and animals.

A heterogenetic effect means that the oil will have a balancing effect on the whole body, rather than just one healing action, unlike
many of today's medications, which can often throw off the body's
equilibrium.

The holistic properties of essential oils enable the body to trigger
its own healing abilities. Just as the plant uses essential oils for its
own survival and reproduction, we borrow from nature to do the
same.

From the Plant to the Bottle

It takes thousands of tons of plant material to steam distill small
amounts of essential oils from the microscopic secretory sacs in
flowers, leaves, roots, bark, and fruit rinds.

Not all plant material is steam distilled either. Citrus oils are cold
pressed from fruits and fine delicate flowers (like jasmine and
rose), going through a solvent extraction process. The essential
oils are not oily, as their name suggests, but they are fat-like, and
volatile substances, which means they absorb well into your skin

and can evaporate quite quickly. Being fats, they will separate in water and float to the surface.

CO_2 extraction is becoming an increasingly popular method to create higher-grade therapeutic oils. This process enables more of the plant's healing compounds to be kept intact rather than destroyed through heat and steam methods.

Distillation is quite an involved process. Once the oils are extracted, they are poured into small amber or blue glass bottles to protect them from UV ray damage. Violet glass bottles are the best form of protection since they block damaging UV rays almost completely, and you will find that the shelf life of your essential oils and remedies will be extended comparatively longer than with amber or blue glass bottles.

Essential Oil Research

Numerous studies are taking place around the globe regarding the efficacy of essential oils for our health (see the bibliography for more details). Here are a few research findings:

- Tea Tree – The most promising new function for this oil is to counter Methicillin-Resistant Staphylococcus aureas (MRSA), the hospital super bug. Hospital MSA-eradication trials using tea tree in creams, ointments and body washes outweigh their traditional chemical counterparts. I have personally witnessed the benefits of tea tree in a hospital in the U.K. when the MRSA bacteria was at its most virulent and my stepfather had been hospitalized. Every one of the patients in the surrounding rooms and beds became infected with the bacteria except for my stepfather who had 0.25 percent solution of tea tree sprayed on the rails of his hospital bed and his hands. Visitors washed their hands with this tea tree blend before and after their visits.

- Tea Tree has also been shown to successfully treat hand warts when applied once daily for twelve days.
- Frankincense - Doctor Hsueh-Kung Lin of the University of Oklahoma commented: "Frankincense oil may represent an inexpensive alternative therapy for patients currently suffering from bladder cancer." According to one study, Frankincense proved to kill cancer cells, ignore normal cell and produce no side effects.
- Lemongrass and Lemon Verbena – proved to be an effective bactericidal against the H Pylori Bacteria.
- Ylang Ylang, Lavender, Marjoram and Neroli – have been shown to control hypertension.
- Thyme and Oregano – show significant results in effectively fighting bacterial throat infections. They are also showing favorable results in treating the Brucellosis bacteria in vitro. This is a very nasty, infectious bacterial disease which has displayed a high resistance to antibiotics. More members of the medical community have turned to plant medicine as a result to combat this particularly stubborn bacteria.

Using Essential Oils for your Health

There are many different methods for using essential oils. Here are the proven main uses:

- Improve your immune system.
- Help you recover from a cold or flu.
- Sooth muscles, aches and pains.

- Clear up skin disorders.
- Help improve women's disorders.
- Improve circulation.
- Stimulate the lymphatic system.
- Calm the nervous system.
- Affect our moods.
- Fragrance our homes.

Combining the benefits of essential oils with tea helps a person to sustain his or her body's natural balance and well-being.

When not to use Essential Oils

Despite being derived from nature, essential oils are very potent. You should always seek professional guidance before using them, especially if any of the points below apply to you:

- Avoid essential oils if you are pregnant.
- Cancer: avoid aniseed and fennel as they may cause hallucinations. For estrogenic cancer, avoid geranium and lavender.
- Hay fever: avoid lavender.
- Allergic to avocado: avoid avocado oil, nuts, and sweet almond.
- If you are taking homeopathic remedies; avoid black pepper, camphor, eucalyptus, peppermint, rosemary, spearmint and tea tree as these may have adverse effects.
- High blood pressure: avoid black pepper, clove, peppermint and rosemary.
- Low blood pressure: avoid prolonged daily use of lavender
- Allergic to the ragweed family: avoid chamomile.
- Epilepsy: avoid camphor, fennel, hyssop and rosemary.

- If you have had an alcoholic drink, avoid an aromatherapy massage. The blend may cause your body to detox too quickly; some oils can cause hallucinations when combined with alcohol.
- Sunbathing: only use the oils at night.

AVOID COMPLETELY: Bitter Almond, Birch, Boldo Leaf, Calamus, Yellow Camphor, Cassia, Cinnamon, Chamomile moroc, Fennel bitter, Horseradish, Mugwort, Pennyroyal, Rue, Sage, Sassafras, Spikenard, Savin, Tagettes, Tansy, Thuja, Turpentine, Wintergreen, Wormwood, Wormseed, Yarrow. These oils are known to contain potent compounds and can be lethal when used in high doses.

Store your essential oils out of sunlight;
away from steam, heat, and children.

Creating a Palette of Color and Fragrance for your Mind, Body and Emotions

"I perhaps owe having become a painter to flowers"
-Claude Monet.

The art of aromatherapy lies in your sense of smell, and the journey it takes you on as you blend individual fragrances to create one single multifaceted aroma. The knowledge, practice, and methods for using essential oils all come together when you are in tune with how an essential oil makes you feel.

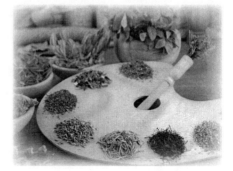

What do you experience when you smell peppermint? Where do your memories take you when you smell rosemary? Who really is the mysterious rose and why is patchouli making you feel so sensuous?

Every essential oil – and there are about 350 of them – has its very own personality. Start by introducing yourself to this great family of healers on a daily basis and you will soon discover their characteristics and the impact they make on your senses, and your physical health. I am so close to each one of them that I almost see them in human form when I am choosing oils specific to my clients' needs. In the beginning work with the oils that really appeal to you, and you will start to build an effective aromatic pharmacy.

As you pick and choose your favorite oils, you will also understand how they affect your blend by the way in which they pour from the bottle. Heavier, resinous oils will take longer to pour, meaning they will create depth and will evaporate slowly, whereas the lighter quicker pouring oils will often give you the mid to top notes of your blend, and evaporate quickly.

Bringing your senses into the mix will truly inspire you and take you to a deeper understanding of the art of aromatherapy. The following pages will give you some guidance notes for nine essential oils: when to use them and how.

Essential Oil Basic Care Kit

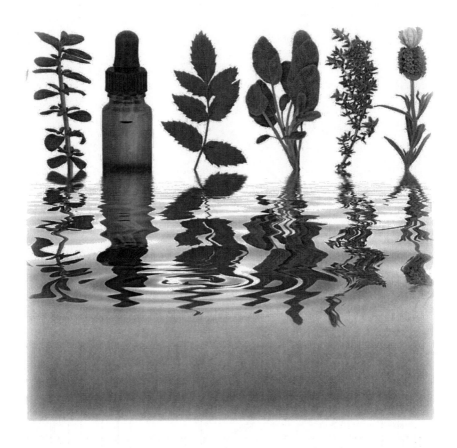

"Hot lavender, mints, savory, marjoram,
The marigold, that goes to bed wi' th' sun
And with him rises weeping. These are flowers
of middle summer ..."
- The Winter's Tale. William Shakespeare

ஜ Bergamot
Citrus *aurantium ssp. Bergamia*

> *- Anti-depressive*
> *- Calming for the body*
> *- Soothes nervous indigestion*

This essential oil may:
-   Help nervous depression.
-   Soothe anxiety.
-   Calm indigestion related to stress, bloating/distension.
-   Encourage feelings of optimism.

Application
- **Digestion:** 25 ml sweet almond oil, 8 drops bergamot, 7 drops lavender. Mix oils together and massage abdomen three times daily.
- **Relaxation:** Use bergaptene-free bergamot essential oil for the bath; add 4 drops to a teaspoon of sweet almond oil to promote relaxation and ease anxiety.
- **Agitation:** Diffuse up to 10 drops in a room diffuser. May stimulate the hypothalamus in the brain to release various regulating and calming neurochemicals.

Blends well with: Lavender, neroli, jasmine, geranium, chamomile roman, coriander, rosemary.
Avoid: Using before going out into the sun.

ஜ **Tea:** Blends well with black tea.

⚜ Chamomile Roman
Anthem *nobilis*

- Calming
- Sedative
- Antispasmodic

This essential oil may:
- Help Rheumatic pain.
- Ease headaches/migraines.
- Reduce insomnia.
- Soothe gas and calm indigestion.
- Release nervous stress.
- Help to relax and avoid the need to be in control.

Application
- **Irritability or Insomnia:** 1-2 drops of chamomile in a teaspoon of sweet almond oil poured into the bath nightly.
- **Headaches:** 1 tablespoon sweet almond oil, 1 drop chamomile, 4 drops lavender. Massage temples and base of neck as needed.
- **Nervous Digestion:** 4 drops of chamomile in 25 ml sweet almond oil. Massage over stomach and liver three times daily.
- **Rheumatic pain:** 6 drops of lavender, 4 drops of chamomile in 25 ml of sweet almond oil; massage over painful area as required.
- **Calm:** Apply 5 drops of chamomile and 6 drops of lavender in a 25 ml spray bottle filled with distilled water. Mist liberally around your head, inhaling deeply.

Blends well with: Bergamot, clary sage, lavender, geranium, jasmine.
Avoid: If you are allergic to the ragweed family.

⚜ **Tea:** Dried Chamomile flowers.

⚛ Eucalyptus
Eucalyptus *globulus*

- Expectorant
- Improves breathing
- Clarifying

This essential oil may help:
- Sinusitis.
- Bronchitis.
- Colds/flu.

- Arthritis.
- Keep insects away.
- Soothe the nerves.

Application
- **Sinusitis:** Add 2 drops of peppermint and a drop of eucalyptus to a bowl of hot water, throw a towel over your head and steam for up to 5 minutes. Splash with cold water to finish. If you have asthma, avoid this technique as it may aggravate it.
- **Bronchitis:** Add 4 drops of eucalyptus, 1 drop of red thyme, 2 drops of oregano, 1 drop of clove, 6 drops of rosemary to 25 ml of sweet almond oil and massage the chest area; front and back; between the shoulder blades; and up towards the neck. Apply twice daily, placing warm compresses over the area after massaging.
- **Immune Tonic:** Add 8 drops of eucalyptus and 4 drops of tea tree to 25 ml sweet almond oil. Massage over thymus and lung area.
- **Calming:** In a room diffuser, add up to 8 drops of eucalyptus for its clarifying effects.

Blends well with: Rosemary, peppermint, marjoram, cedarwood, lemon.
Avoid: With high blood pressure.

✂ **Tea:** Peppermint

❦ Geranium
Pelargonium *graveloens*

- For Skincare

- Hormones

This essential oil may help:
- Balance sensitive, dry or mature skin.
- Infertility.

- PMS, Menopause.
- Nerve, joint and facial neuralgia.
- Work-related stress.

Application
- **PMS & Menopause:** Add 5 drops geranium, 6 drops clary sage and 4 drops lavender to 30 ml of sweet almond oil. Use ½ capful in bath nightly or as a body oil after showering, paying attention to areas behind the knees, wrists, and elbow creases.
- **Infertility (stress induced):** Add 7 drops geranium, 3 drops clary sage, 2 drops ylang ylang, 4 drops lavender, and 1 drop patchouli to 25 ml sweet almond oil. Massage into lower abdomen and pelvis three times daily. Stop during period. If estrogen is dominating over progesterone, reduce geranium to 2 drops, increase clary sage to 5 drops.
- **Skincare:** Add 12 drops of geranium and 4 drops of lavender to 30 ml jojoba oil. Gently massage into the face nightly after cleansing. Will smooth and tone the skin.
- **Work-related stress:** Add 5 drops geranium, and 7 drops lavender to a 25 ml spray bottle filled with distilled water. Mist liberally around your head, inhaling deeply.

Blends well with: Sandalwood, jasmine, neroli, bergamot, patchouli, lavender, citrus oils.

❦ **Tea:** None

⚘ Grapefruit
Citrus paradisis

- Purifying
- Cooling
- Lymphatic stimulant

This essential oil may help:

- Cellulite.
- Oedema.
- Lose weight.
- Oily Skin.

- Depression.
- Clear frustration.
- Improve self-esteem.

Application

- **Cellulitis & Weight Loss:** 16 oz Epsom salts – add 30 drops Grapefruit, 16 drops Rosemary, 4 drops Juniper, 2 teaspoons sweet almond oil. Mix together and use 2 table-spoons in bath three times a week.
- **Comfort Eating/Mood Lift:** 100 ml distilled water in spray bottle, add 90 drops Grapefruit. Spray liberally around head and into hands. May release "feel good" neurochemicals from the brain to prevent over-eating and boost self-esteem.

Blends well with: Bergamot, lavender, rosemary, juniper, cypress, spice oils.

Avoid: If you are taking medications, check with your health care practitioner before using grapefruit.

⚘ **Tea:** Add a drop of grapefruit oil to 1 teaspoon of green tea.

✾ Lavender
Lavandula *angustifolia*

- Calming
- For Insomnia
- May be used directly on the skin without blending

This essential oil may help:

- Arthritis and muscular aches.
- Burns, bruises, sprains.
- Sunburn.
- Radiation burns.
- High blood pressure.

- Irregular heart beat.
- Insomnia.
- Anxiety.
- Migraines/headaches.
- Calm nerves and reduce stress.

Application

- **Calm and relax:** May release serotonin when inhaled to relax and calm the nervous system.
- **Radiation Burns:** Add 25 drops lavender and 8 drops frankincense to a 50 ml distilled water spray bottle; mist radiated area to reduce burning. Can also use same blend with jojoba gel (25 ml) and apply. Use the night before, and following treatment. Do not use on the day of radiation.
- **Insomnia:** 1 drop on each temple, under nose, on chest & pillows nightly.
- **Skin Care:** Clean congested skin by steaming with 3 drops of lavender and 2 drops lemon. Drape a towel over your head and steam your face over a sink filled with hot water for five minutes.
- **Muscular aches:** 25 ml sweet almond oil, 8 drops lavender, 3 drops rosemary and 1 drop peppermint. Massage area. (Avoid rosemary if you have high blood pressure.)

Blends well with most essential oils.

✿ **Tea:** Dried loose lavender tea.

⚜ Peppermint
Mentha piperita

- Analgesic
- Decongests
- For Nausea
- Awakens

This essential oil may help:
- Migraines/headaches
- Sciatica and pain
- Indigestion and nausea
- Repel mosquitoes
- Gas
- Sinuses (also see Eucalyptus)
- Mental tiredness
- Improve Concentration

Application
- **Headaches/Migraines:** Add 3 drops of peppermint and 5 drops of lavender to 10 ml of sweet almond carrier oil; apply to temples, and back of neck. Avoid if your migraine makes you intolerant to smells.
- **Sciatica/Pain:** Add 4 drops of peppermint to 10 ml of sweet almond carrier oil and apply to affected area as required.
- **Indigestion and nausea:** Massage the stomach area with the same blend as for sciatica and inhale the oil to reduce nausea.
- **Mental tiredness**: Add 4 drops of peppermint to an electric room diffuser or 8 drops to a candle diffuser's bowl filled with warm water.
- **Insect repellant:** Use the blend for mental tiredness in a diffuser outside;, mixed with 10 drops of lemongrass, 3 drops of clove and 4 drops of rosemary.

Blends well with: Lavender, eucalyptus, rosemary, lemongrass, marjoram, rosemary.
Avoid: With high blood pressure

⚜ **Tea:** Peppermint.

✿ Tea Tree
Melaleuca alternifolia

- Immune System
- Disinfectant
- Empowerment
- May be used directly on the skin without diluting

This essential oil may help:

- Athlete's foot.
- Skin infections.
- Candida.
- Cold/Flu/Sore throat.
- Cold sores.
- Bronchitis.
- Strengthen resistance to disease.
- Build confidence.

Application

- **Immune System:** Add 12 drops of tea tree oil to 25 ml sweet almond oil and massage body after showering with oil, daily.
- **Disinfectant:** Use as a hand sanitizer directly on the skin. You can also add 15 drops of tea tree to 25 ml of distilled water in a small spray bottle and disinfect areas of public use.
- **Athlete's foot:** Apply 2 drops of tea tree directly to affected area, three times daily.
- **Ingrown nail infection:** Add 15 drops of tea tree, 3 drops thyme, 2 drops oregano, and 1 drop myrrh to 25 ml of sweet almond oil or jojoba gel. Apply twice daily.
- **Candida:** Apply a drop of tea tree on your tooth brush twice daily when brushing teeth to help clear candida in the mouth. Use the immune system blend above and add one cap to a nightly bath for vaginal yeast infections.

Blends well with: Lavender, myrrh, marjoram, rosemary, lemon, eucalyptus.

✿ **Tea:** *Matcha*

☘ Ylang Ylang
Cananga odorata

- For High Blood Pressure
- Calming
- Palpitations

This essential may help:
- Regulate blood pressure.
- Calm palpitations.
- Calm the nervous system.
- Boost sensuality.

Application
- **Blood pressure regulator**: Add 15 drops of lavender and 10 drops of ylang ylang to 50 ml of sweet almond oil. Massage into the chest twice daily. Check with your health care practitioner before using.
- **Sensuality:** To reconnect to feelings of intimacy or sensuality add 4 drops of ylang ylang, 1 drop of patchouli, and 2 drops of geranium rose to 25 ml of sweet almond oil. Use one capful in the bath nightly or as a massage oil.

Blends well with: Lavender, rose, geranium, bergamot, rose, vanilla, vetiver.

☙ **Tea:** Rose and lavender tea, white tea, hibiscus tea.

The Body Beautiful and Essential Oils

You can use essential oils to help with muscular aches and pains, headaches, sinus congestion, stomachaches, and many types of physical ailments. Here is why:

When you apply essential oils to your skin, they need to be diluted in a carrier oil like sweet almond or jojoba (otherwise they may irritate the skin). The oil molecules penetrate directly into your bloodstream, bypassing the digestive system, having a more immediate effect on body aches and ailments.

The oils are easily absorbed by the skin and can linger in your body for up to seven hours before they are expelled.

On-going research suggests that a smaller dosage of essential oil is more effective on the body. When too many drops are used, this can overwhelm any physiological effect; counteracting the benefit of the oil.

The Best Method For Applying Oils to Your Skin:

The quickest method is in the bath where the oils penetrate the open pores of your skin as you relax.

Alternatively, massaging the oils over your whole body just after showering - while your skin is warm - will also help absorption.

Essential oils diluted in a carrier oil like sweet almond or apricot kernel oil can be massaged under the armpits, the soles of the feet, inside the wrists, behind knees as well as the creases of the elbows for optimum absorption.

The toughest places for oils to be absorbed are on your abdomen, legs, and buttocks

Creating your Massage or Bath Blend

To create your essential oil blend, choose up to three essential oils from the same family such as the herb family: rosemary, marjoram and lemon balm; or flowers: lavender, geranium and rose. When you are just starting out I suggest just choosing one, see the Basic Care Kit for further details.

The best way to start is to use one essential oil and blend it in a blue or violet glass bottle, a 1 oz/30 ml size will last you about five baths or five full body massages for use after showering.

Create a clean space in your kitchen for blending and make certain there are no animals nearby; and plenty of ventilation. The tools you use to mix the oils now become part of your aromatherapy tool kit and are not shared with your everyday cooking utensils.

Blending guide for a bath/massage oil

1. Fill a 30 ml bottle with sweet almond oil – a carrier oil.
2. To calculate the number of essential oil drops required, divide the quantity of fluid in the bottle by two.
3. Therefore, a 30 ml bottle of carrier oil will require 15 drops total of essential oil. If you have sensitive skin, divide by four , so that is approximately six drops of oil.
4. Choose one essential oil from the Basic Care Kit that works for you and add 15 drops to the bottle of sweet almond oil. If you are combining two or three essential oils, break down the number of drops for each oil so that the total number of drops reaches 15.

5. For example a blend of three oils could be: 8 drops of lavender, 3 drops of geranium, 4 drops of rose.

Keep a recipe book or card index of the blends you create and your reaction to them, including how you feel, and whether the oils helped your health situation.

6. Label your oil blend.
7. Use one capful per bath and pour the oil into the water just before getting in as the aromatic molecules will dissipate quickly in the hot water, and you want to enjoy the fragrance for as long as you can. Alternatively, use the oil to massage onto your body after showering or have someone massage you!

Oils that irritate the skin:

Be aware that when you blend essential oils for the bath, some of them can redden the skin or make you itch. If you feel these sensations or have breathing difficulties, get out of the bath swiftly and shower it off with cold water. Oils you definitely want to avoid in the bath are the following:

- Angelica
- Anise
- Basil
- Camphor
- Cinnamon
- Citronella
- Citrus
- Clove
- Cumin
- Lemongrass
- Melissa
- Nutmeg
- Peppermint
- Thyme

Testing for skin sensitivity:

Before using essential oils, you can perform a skin sensitivity test by adding one drop of essential oil to a teaspoon of sweet almond carrier oil, and then testing it on the inside of your arm. If redness or itching occurs, avoid that particular essential oil.

The Power of Fragrance
on Your Senses

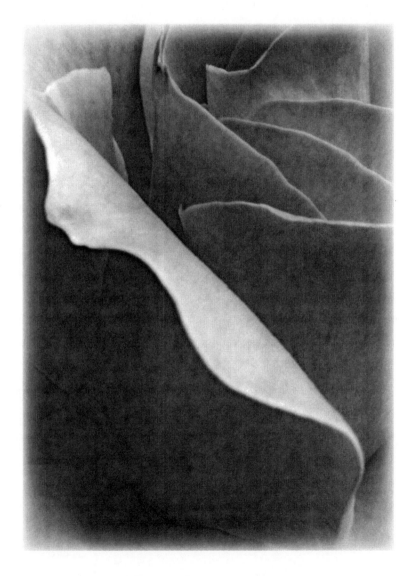

"The world is a rose; smell it and pass it to your friends."
Persian Proverb

Aroma and Your Emotions

"Every plant and flower has its own signature aroma, calling us with a secret language that defies conscious translation, but somehow we feel changed after sensing it."
- Nicola

Smell has been one of the last senses to be explored by the scientific community. How it affects our emotions and enhances our sense of taste is still being studied.

Through smell, we connect to long lost memories; we subconsciously identify people, and are attracted (or not) through their smell.

Our noses are fine pieces of technical engineering with an ability to identify up to 10,000 different odors. We have about 50 million receptors in our noses that transmit odors as electric impulses to the olfactory bulb in the brain. From here, the electric impulses are sent to the amygdala (this stores and releases emotional trauma), and they then carry onto the limbic system (the oldest part of the brain), which distributes the impulses to other parts of the brain controlling heart rate, blood pressure, breathing, memory, stress and hormones.

Different aromas will bring about different benefits for our bodies and psyches by stimulating or calming us. The aroma of a lavender bush on a warm summer's evening may remind you of your grandmother, and the good times you had with her. Perhaps the smell of vanilla reminds you of your mother baking cakes in the kitchen; of being cared for and feeling safe.

Aroma and your Thoughts

The aroma of essential oils, tea or any fragrance appear to impact our senses and bodies, helping to stimulate, relax or balance us.

Through smell we begin to feel more uplifted, calmed or invigorated and because we feel good, we start to think differently, perhaps more positively, becoming increasingly aware that there may be certain negative thoughts we like to keep replaying in our brains that are actually destructive to our health and well-being.

You see, everything you think affects your physical body.

Research in pyschoneuroimmunology, the study of the intrinsic connection between the mind and and the body, has continued to expand in western medicine.

Negative thoughts can release damaging neurochemicals, putting the body under stress and creating a disease. When we are able to switch that thought to a positive one, a change may occur in our health and well-being.

Using teas and essential oils daily to relax and calm you will benefit your mental, emotional and physical states.

Smell to Relax

At the Sense of Smell Institute at Wesleyen University, the aroma of lavender was rigorously tested for its effect on night time sleep and was found to improve sleep in men, and even more so for women.

The Wheeling Jesuit University also discovered in tests that the scent of jasmine improved the sleep quality of participants. These individuals who performed cognitive tests more rapidly than those who inhaled lavender. In addition, these participants were unaware of breathing the aroma of jasmine during their sleep, thus revealing that human bodies respond to odors even when they are unconscious of them.

Smell to Stay Awake

Additional research has shown that smelling an essential oil affects the adrenal system via the sympathetic nervous system. Black pepper can increase adrenaline, helping us to stay alert, while rose decreases adrenaline levels.

Reach for a Better Mood through Aroma

The following tables give categories of mood enhancing essential oils established by Robert Tisserand, a celebrated aromatherapist from England, one of the first to spread the word about aromatherapy and its uses. Thanks to him and many other leaders in the field, aromatherapy has become what it has today.

I have added additional oils to his original tables, following positive feedback from my clients. They used the power of aroma to help shift their moods that also helped to change the "energy" or mood in their living and working environments.

Our emotional well-being impacts the energy of our homes by 50 percent. The location, direction and structure of the home will also impact our well-being as per the principles of Feng Shui, which is the Chinese art of balancing vital energies in an environment to promote a balanced flow of energy, health and prosperity.

By using essential oils for your emotional well-being, you will feel calmer, happier and more peaceful, thereby helping others around you to feel the same. You will notice how your home will become more inviting and relaxing.

The Power of Smell to Improve Your Mood

1. Aphrodisiac Oils

For: Shyness, Impotence, Frigidity, Disconnection from your true self.

Essential Oil	1 fl oz Massage Oil No. of drops	1 fl oz Spray No. of drops	4 fl oz Spray No. of drops
Clary Sage	5–8	8–10	20–25
Geranium	6	8	25–30
Jasmine	4	5	18
Patchouli	4	5	15
Vetiver	3	5	15
Ylang Ylang	4	5	15

) (

2. Euphoric Oils

For: Moodiness, lack of confidence, depression, sadness.

Essential Oil	1 fl oz Massage Oil No. of Drops	1 fl oz Spray No. of Drops	4 fl oz Spray No. of Drops
Bergamot	10	13	35–40
Clary Sage	5–8	8–10	25–30
Grapefruit	15	15–18	40
Jasmine	4	5	18
Rose Otto	4	5–6	18–20

3. Invigorating & Creativity Oils

For: Boosting motivation, release from lethargy and immune deficiency.

Essential Oils	1 fl oz Massage Oil No. of Drops	1 fl oz Spray No. of Drops	4 fl oz Spray No. of Drops
Cardamon	3	5	15
Juniper	4	6	25
Lemongrass	3	6	15
Rosemary	8	12	30

( ) ( )

4. Memory/Mental Stimulating Oils

For: Mental fatigue, poor concentration, poor memory.

Essential Oils	1 fl oz Massage Oil No. of Drops	1 fl oz Spray No. of Drops	4 fl oz Spray No. of Drops
Black Pepper	4	9	20 – 36
Lemon	15	15-18	40
Peppermint	5	10	30-40
Rosemary	8	12	30

5. Regulating Oils

For: Anxiety, Depression, Mood swings.

Essential Oils	1 fl oz Massage Oil No. of Drops	1 fl oz Spray No. of Drops	4 fl oz Spray No. of Drops
Bergamot	10	13	35-40
Frankincense	8	12	40-45
Geranium	6	8	25-30
Rosewood	6-8	15	40

6. Sedative Oils

For: Anxiety, Stress, Hypertension, Insomnia, Anger, Irritability.

Essential Oils	1 fl oz Massage Oil No. of Drops	1 fl oz Spray No. of Drops	4 fl oz Spray No. of Drops
Roman Chamomile	4	8	30
Lavender	15	18-20	55
Marjoram	8	18-20	35-45
Peru Balsam	5	10	30
Orange Blossom	8	15	40
Ylang Ylang	4	5	15
Sandalwood	4	5	15

Mood Balancing Tools For Your Environment

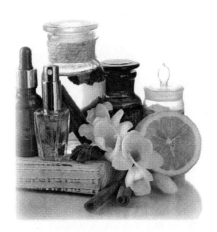

The oils shown on the tables can be used in the following ways to change your mood.

• Electric/Candle Diffuser

To maintain a lovely scent and a feeling of well-being through-out your home or office, choose an essential oil from the chart, and decide whether you are going to use an electric diffuser that blows cold air through the essential oil, or a candle burner that gently warms the oils in a small bowl of water sitting atop a candle holder.

An electric diffuser is safer since it can be left on for 15 minutes per hour. Any longer than that and you may find it gives you a headache, or unable to smell the blend.

• Room or Body Atomizer

To uplift or calm your mood, a room or body atomizer is a great way to release the essential molecules into the air. Breath deeply for an optimum effect.

How to Make a Room Spray/Body Atomizer

For a pocket-size spray, use a 1 fl oz blue or amber glass bottle with a spray cap. Fill this with distilled water, and add your oils, up to

15 drops. Start with one or two drops and then build the blend from there, pausing to smell to check you like it.

For a larger room spray to clean and clear the air, take a larger 4 fl oz glass bottle with spray cap, fill with distilled water and then add up to 50 drops of your chosen oil or oils..

Remember, if you choose a combination of oils, then the *total* number should add up to 50 drops for a 4 fl oz bottle, which is about 100 ml.

Avoid using plastic sprayers as the essential oils will destroy the bottle; they are potent and can mangle plastic if they are in the bottle for too long a period.

How to Use the Sprays

For your personal body mist, liberally mist your aromatic creation around your head and into your hands, breathing deeply to help shift your mood. Some of the heavier oils may leave a lingering fragrance; the lighter oils will dissipate after a few seconds.

For the room mist, spray the room liberally, sending your aromatic molecules into closets, bathrooms and the kitchen to freshen and clear the atmosphere. The molecules will also set to work, providing an antibacterial and possibly antiviral environment.

• Massage/Bath Oil Blend

See the Body Beautiful section on how to make a massage/bath blend on page 145.

A Tea Break for your Soul

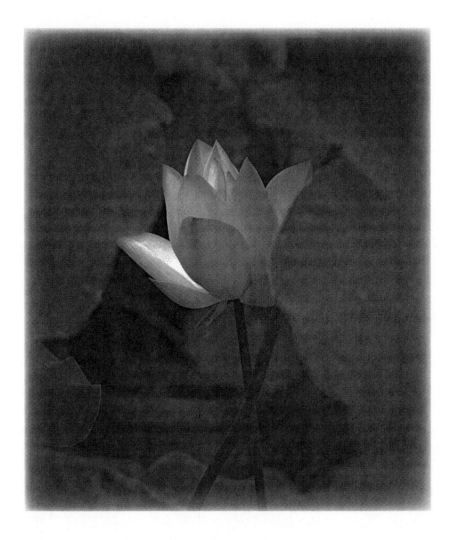

"Life is short, make it sweet."
-Sri Kaleshwar

The Power of Tea for Inner Contemplation and Inspiration

> *"Your soul is that inner feeling of being inspired to follow your dreams and follow the beat of your own drum."*
> *- Nicola*

For some individuals, living life according to the dictates of one's soul means being authentic and genuine; practicing random acts of kindness; compassion, being of service; making others happy; seeing life from a more expanded place, and perhaps observing your role in life and why you are here.

Some see it as living continuously from a heart-based wisdom, trusting the heart's direction and following its lead; and coming from a place of forgiveness.

In truth, it is all of these plus many more directives that our soul sends us daily to help us create our lives consciously; ultimately culminating in understanding that we ourselves are already living in our greatness and perfection, if we could all but see it. The soul is the Divine self, it is our true consciousness, without ego and illusion.

Tea - A Meditation for your Soul

Quietness and meditation with a cup of tea helps us to observe our lives. We don't necessarily need to sit in a dark quiet corner with a candle every day to meditate, although it can help avoid distractions!

> *The simple art and pleasure of making and pouring your chosen tea means you are taking care of yourself. A moment in time where it really is all about you and having a moment to just be.*

The more quiet we become, the greater the opportunity we have to "listen" to that small inner voice that always speaks the truth.

Some of us will ignore it while our lower minds give excuses for not taking that much needed vacation; visiting family, or spending more time with friends because of work, or "things" that need to be done at home.

Others may take a sip of tea to help them make a final decision on the next phase of their life's journey. Some will be inspired to create and bring out their true magic.

Your tea break may bring you many things, perhaps life changing, or to appreciate and enjoy the more subtle pleasures of life. It will definitely give you a window of time to just savor and treasure the moment with your favorite cup of tea.

Indeed, the traditional "tea break" can be taken to an even deeper level by using the time to tap into your creativity by drinking powdered *matcha* green tea to aid in relaxation and meditation for 10 minutes or a few hours, following the ancient tradition of the Zen Buddhist monks who use *matcha* for long periods of focus, relaxation and Divine inspiration.

Tea as Medicine for your Life-force

As you are making your cup of tea, you may not be aware that you are also handling subtle energies contained within your tea and essential oils. These subtle energies are the life-force of the plant.

In traditional Chinese medicine, you will hear of the invisible energy life-force called *Qi;* known as *Ki* in Japanese, and *Prana* in Sanskrit. They all refer to the energy that animates every living thing on the planet. *Qi* exists as a form of electricity generated through our cells and also around us. The sun, for example, energizes the plants with light, thereby stimulating growth. The sun's rays are converted into energy, creating electricity in the plant's cells, which then create a life-force or field around the plant called a biofield or magnetic field. We as humans also possess the same ability.

Fresh herbal teas picked straight from their plant source will have a greater "energy" or life-force than dried tea leaves. The same applies to essential oils extracted from plants and grown without pesticides or chemicals.

We are subconsciously affected by the life-force in our food and drinks. Chemically- treated teas and food drain our bodies of vital energies and we flourish when we ingest foods that possess vitality; we look better and feel better. The energy of these foods also affects our "subtle bodies" and our power-storing energy centers.

Ancient traditions talk of our subtle bodies, and unlike Western medicine, the subtle energy body (a non-visible imprint of your physical body that surrounds you), and the physical body are seen as one, and not separated. Indeed, Eastern medicine recognizes that illness can actually originate in the subconscious, or subtle energy body.

Chakras, Teas and Essential Oils Unite

The Chakras are a powerful energy system understood by Ayurvedic healers for thousands of years, and believed to balance the body's health and emotional well-being.

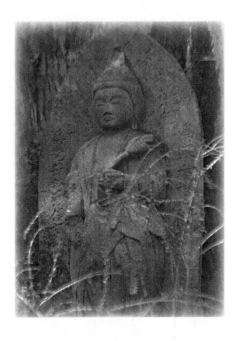

The word chakra means "spinning wheel of energy/ light," and each one receives and releases energy from nature. There are seven key chakras: the first one begins at the base of the spinal column, followed up the spine by the others to end just above the crown. Each one has its own unique function; just like a well-oiled clock, they interact as a whole and determine - among many things - how we are feeling; how we react to situations; how we seek fulfillment in this lifetime, and how present and confident we are.

There is an additional chakra called the eighth or soul chakra hovering about 12 inches above our heads like a halo of light radiating with strands of light to connect us to a higher wisdom and nature.

The chakra system can be compared to our signpost in life. For example, if we are having difficulty expressing our needs, or our truth, it can be said that there is a stagnation of energy in the throat chakra, and sometimes a physical disease in the throat may occur because of our fear or inability to express what we feel.

Each chakra represents different states of our personality, and when one is out of balance we will be either overly reactive, or unresponsive to emotional situations. We can use essential oils and teas to help us develop a deeper awareness of ourselves; fine-tune our reactions, our attitudes, how we interact, and have a greater sense of who we are and perhaps what we want to change or improve about ourselves.

The following pages will give an overview of chakra meanings, and the essential oils and teas to use with each chakra. There are directions after the tables , which will show you how to choose the oil and tea specific for your energy needs.

**7th Chakra – Crown – I am connected. I trust.
Divine inspiration. Self-realization.**

Located: Top of the head and impacts the brain – cerebral cortex, pineal gland.

🕉 *Essential Oils:*

- Pink or white lotus – for feeling at one with the universe.
- Frankincense – for spiritual consciousness.
- Myrrh – uniting the spiritual and physical bodies.
- Sandalwood – for expanding your consciousness and connecting with your role in this lifetime.

🍃 *Tea: Matcha*

6th Chakra - 3rd eye – I see the truth. Intuition.

Located: On the forehead between the eyebrows; impacts the eyes, sinuses, pituitary gland and hypothalamus..

Essential Oils:

- Clary Sage – for intuition.
- Sandalwood – for surrender.
- Jasmine – for inspiration.

Tea: Jasmine. Or add 1 drop of jasmine oil to a folded square of tissue an dplace in a canister that holds a tbsp of green tea. Store for a couple of days before using. The tea will become infused with the fragrance of jasmine.

5th Chakra- Throat – I communicate clearly. I express creatively.

Located: At the throat; impacts the throat, jaw, mouth, ears, shoulders and thyroid.

Essential Oils:

- Lavender- for clear/calm expression/releasing self-consciousness.
- Cedarwood – holding words/expressions firm.
- German Chamomile – calm control.

Tea: Lavender

4th Chakra - Heart – I love myself. Unconditional love for others. Kindness to self and others. Forgiveness.

Located: At the heart; impacts the heart, lungs, shoulders, arms, hands and thymus.

🕯 *Essential Oils:*

- Rose – restores trust, warmth and helps overcome grief.
- Neroli – reassurance.
- Palma Rosa – opens the heart.

🍵 *Tea:* Rose and/or green, hibiscus, *matcha.*

3rd Chakra - Solar Plexus – I am. Staying true to your nature with a healthy relationship to personal power.

Located: At the stomach area just under the rib cage; impacts the liver, stomach, pancreas, gallbladder and intestines.

🕯 *Essential Oils:*

- Chamomile Roman – releases tension.
- Grapefruit – purifies and empowers.
- Rosemary – builds self worth.
- Lemon – clears fear and heat.

🍵 *Tea:* Black with added lemon or grapefruit oil, *oolong* with lemon, or green tea with lemon or grapefruit oil.

2nd Chakra – Navel – Place of self. I feel. I am creatively active.

Located: Four finger-widths below the navel; impacts the kidneys, bladder, sex organs, hips, sacrum and adrenals.

🕉 *Essential Oils:*

- Patchouli – reawakens the senses.

- *Ylang Ylang* – releases sexuality blocks, fear.

- Geranium – reconnects to intimacy, trust.

🌱 *Tea:* Ginger, mint tea, black or chai.

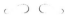

**1st Chakra - Root – I am grounded and centered.
Abundant. I am safe.**

Located: In the pelvis; impacts the bones, feet, legs, knees, perineum, coccyx and adrenal glands.

🕉 *Essential Oils:*

- Vetiver – centers and grounds.

- Marjoram – nourishes, nurtures and strengthens.

- Myrrh – reconnects you to your physical body.

- Cinnamon – warms and encourages participation in life.

🌱 *Tea:* Rooibus with cinnamon, clove and cardamom added. Black tea, chai, pomegranate.

Directions for Choosing and Using Essential Oils for the Chakras

How are you feeling today? Perhaps life has created a feeling of being overwhelmed or scattered. If this is the case, then try sipping on a *rooibos* or chai to energize your root chakra and pick the essential oil of vetiver to ground and reconnect.

Once you have asked yourself this question choose a tea and essential oil from one of the chakra tables that best suits your mood.

To use the essential oils for a bath or body blend, add 2-3 drops of your oil to a teaspoon of sweet almond oil and use some in the bath, or use as a massage oil over the relevant chakra on your body, daily.

If you prefer, you can use the essential oils to stimulate your senses and balance the chakras through your sense of smell. Add up to 15 drops of your chosen essential oil to a 1 fl oz blue glass bottle filled with distilled water. Spray liberally around your head and body, inhaling deeply throughout the day.

Continue with your chosen essential oil and tea until you feel a difference within yourself, i.e. more confident, grounded or creative.

To further benefit from the vibrational quality of the oil you may also want to fragrance your home or office. You can do this by adding up to 8 drops of your chosen essential to a room diffuser.

The Perfume Artisan –
Turning Tea into Perfume

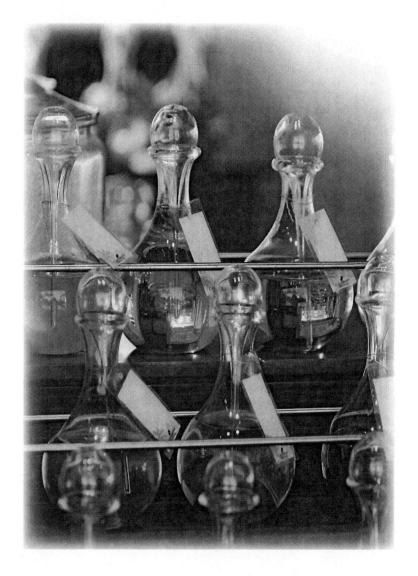

"Perfumes are the feelings of flowers."
-Heinrich Heine

Tea becomes Perfume

A beautifully fragranced leftover tea can be transformed into a cologne or perfume. Discover your untapped talents as a perfume artisan with your ability to make natural aromatic perfume blends with tea. Teas that work best for perfumes are white, green or herbal tea.

The quality of tea doesn't matter in this instance and you can either make a fresh batch of tea for your perfume, using a tea bag, or use the leftover tea from the pot you didn't finish. You can also pick a handful of fresh herbs from the garden to use as a tea base for your perfume.

You will discover that tea will add more depth to your blend and will be better for your skin compared to the harsh chemicals found in commercial perfumes.

Equipment you will need:

- 1 fl oz clean blue glass bottles with either a sprayer or roller ball cap. Pretty vintage bottles will work, but your essential oils may deteriorate more quickly.
- Glass jug or cafetière.
- Green, white or herbal tea. Steeped and cooled.
- Essential oils.
- Vodka.
- Labels to give your perfume a name and date.
- A well-ventilated area.
- A notebook to keep your fragrance recipes

Some Notes for the Perfume Artisan

You will see that I have used vodka in the perfume recipes to extend the fragrance of the essential oils. If you prefer not to use vodka, your perfume may not linger as long on your skin.

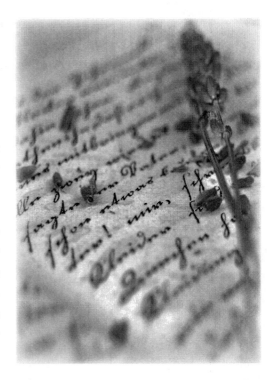

However, you can use heavier oils for a longer lasting fragrance. The heavier, thicker (viscous) essential oils are often darker and slower to pour from the bottle. These are less volatile (slower to evaporate) while the lighter, less viscous oils, such as citrus, are orange, green or yellow in color and evaporate more quickly.

When you blend a mix of heavier and lighter oils, the heavier oils (known as fixatives) will help hold the lighter oils (citrus, for example) to last longer on the skin.

In the world of perfume, we like to refer to essential oils as having "notes." This helps us to categorize the heavier oils from the lighter oils.

The Base Notes – the Healers
The note that lasts the longest in the fragrance is usually a fixative oil: a heavier, more viscous oil, and will make up one to five percent of the blend. They have a strong therapeutic action and will have the lowest evaporation rate. These might be vetiver, sandalwood, myrrh, benzoin, peru balsam, clary sage, and patchouli.

The Mid-Notes – the Feelers
The notes that have cleaner, sharper aromas are the dominant oils, which make up 50-80 percent of the blend. Mid-notes help us connect to our emotions. The oils in this category might be geranium, lavender, and chamomile roman.

The Top Notes – the Sensers
These are the light notes that give the momentary introduction to the blend and help us "come to our senses," so to speak. They will make up 10 percent of the blend and will include oils of citrus, needle, and bergamot.

Create Your Signature Scent

Here are the typical perfumes you can create, depending on your taste, or smell. Be sure to stop and smell your concoction every step of the way and feel free to add more or fewer drops so that the fragrance truly becomes your very own.

- *Green/Grass:* Fresh and invigorating; using evergreen oils such as Cedarwood, Juniper Berry, Pine, Fir and adding some Lavender and a hint of Citrus.

For the blend:
1 fl oz /30 ml green tea – one tea bag or 1 tsp of green tea
1 drop of fir
3 drops of cedarwood
5 drops of lavender
4 drops lemon
4 drops of vodka
1 blue glass bottle with sprayer

Directions
1. Make the green tea in a jug or cafetière with 1 fl oz of boiling water and allow the tea to steep and cool for at least 1 hour.
2. Stir the tea, remove the tea bag and strain the tea into the bottle, add the vodka. Shake well.
3. Gradually add the essential oils to the tea, smelling as you go to check the fragrance. Shake well when finished. Label. Refrigerate for a couple of days before using.

- *Citrus:* Light, fresh and stimulating citrus oils make up the bulk of the perfume with some floral notes added like Lavender, Geranium and Rose.

For the blend:
1 fl.oz /30 ml (one handful of fresh lemon balm) or lemon tea
8 drops of bergamot
4 drops of lavender
3 drops of geranium
4 drops of vodka
1 blue glass bottle with sprayer

Directions
1. Make the lemon balm tea in a jug or cafetière with 1 fl oz of boiling water; allow the tea to steep and cool for at least 2 hours. Alternatively, take 3 slices of lemon and pour boiling water over them and steep for 10 minutes, allow to cool.
2. Stir the tea, strain into the bottle and add the vodka. Shake well.
3. Gradually add the essential oils to the tea, smelling as you go to check the fragrance. Shake well when finished. Label. Refrigerate for a couple of days before using.

- *Floral:* Very feminine using flower oils such as Lavender, Neroli, Rose, Jasmine and *Ylang Ylang.* The perfume can be made with just one of these or a blend.

For the blend:
1 fl oz /30 ml lavender tea made with 2 tsp dried lavender
4 drops of rose
5 drops of bergamot
1 drop of jasmine
4 drops lavender
4 drops of vodka
1 blue glass bottle with sprayer

Directions
1. Make the dried lavender tea in a jug or cafetière with 1 fl oz of boiling water and allow the tea to steep and cool for at least 2 hours.
2. Stir the tea and strain into the bottle and add the vodka. Shake well.
3. Gradually add the essential oils to the tea, smelling as you go to check the fragrance and shaking each time. Shake well when finished. Label. Refrigerate for a couple of days before using.

- *Chypre:* A green fragrance from above blended with floral and citrus touches, and can include Patchouli, Oakmoss, Bergamot, Sandalwood and have a woody, mossy fragrance.

For the blend:
1 fl oz /30 ml chamomile tea made with 1 tea bag or a handful of fresh flowers
1 drop of chamomile roman
1 drop of patchouli
2 drops jasmine
5 drops of bergamot
4 drops of vodka
1 blue glass bottle with sprayer

Directions
1. Make the dried lavender tea in a jug or cafetière with 1 fl oz of boiling water and allow the tea to steep and cool for at least 2 hours.
2. Stir, strain the tea into the bottle and add the vodka. Shake well.
3. Gradually add the essential oils to the tea smelling as you go to check the fragrance shaking each time. Shake well when finished. Label. Refrigerate for a couple of days before using.

- *Oriental:* Mysterious, warm and enticing, these perfumes are heavier and long- lasting. Essential oils such as Patchouli, Sandalwood, Vetiver, Balsam, Ginger are used with Jasmine for a more feminine fragrance, or Clary Sage for a masculine touch.

For the blend:
1 fl oz /30 ml ginger tea
1 drop of vetiver
3 drops of sandalwood
2 drops of jasmine
1 drop of ginger
4 drops of vodka
1 blue glass bottle with sprayer

Directions
1. Make the ginger tea by slicing 5 slices of fresh ginger and adding 1 fl oz of boiling water. Allow the tea to steep and cool for at least 2 hours. You can also replace the fresh ginger with one ginger tea bag and follow the same directions.
2. Stir and strain into the bottle and add the vodka. Shake well.
3. Gradually add the essential oils to the tea, smelling as you go to check the fragrance, shaking each time. Shake well when finished. Label. Refrigerate for a couple of days before using.

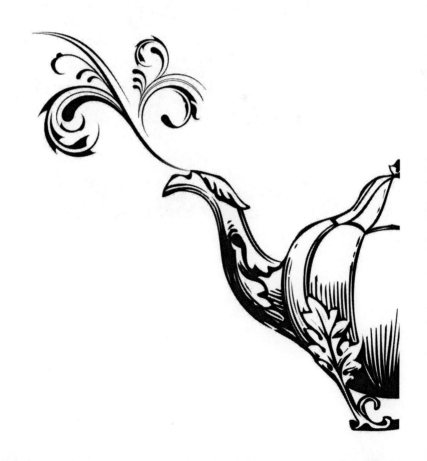

Tea Remedies and Aromatic Elixirs
For Vibrant, Natural, Revitalizing Skincare

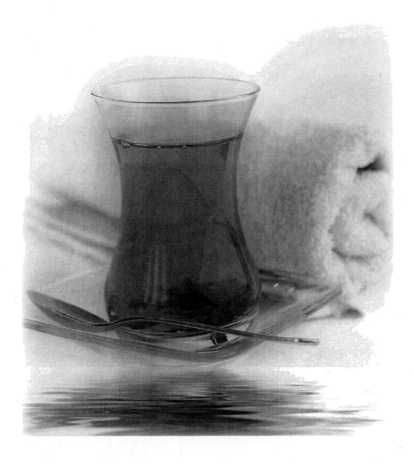

"The earth laughs in flowers."
- Emerson

Steam, Tone, Hydrate and Moisturize

Using tea and essential oils to promote youthful skin tone and good health is a natural approach for taking care of yourself; it's also easy and cost effective to do.

Drinking tea as part of your beauty regime is so simple, its crazy good! With just one cup of green, *matcha*, white or *oolong* tea each day, you are already flooding your body with antioxidants that will improve your skin's elasticity.

The *Journal of Nutrition* recently reported that *"consumption of green tea compounds helps support improvement in women's skin elasticity."* There you have it so let's have some fun.

> *The best teas for your beauty regime are; Green, White, Matcha, Pu'erh, Rooibus, Hibiscus, Pomegranate.*
>
> If you are caffeine-sensitive make your green teas very weak and drink only 1-2 cups a day.

Your Spa Day

Have a spa day for yourself, or invite friends over for a time to kick back and rejuvenate; either way you are sure to benefit from it. Serve hot or iced teas, a tea cocktail from the cocktail section, or a traditional English tea with bite-size sandwiches.

I suggest each guest makes one or two skincare products for the rest of the group to share from the remedies on the following pages. As the hostess, you will need to get a little organized beforehand, supplying teas and bottles. Add to the fun by inviting each of your guests to bring their own teapot and strainer, or cafetière (ideal for pressing the teas/herbs).

Before your guests arrive, create your relaxing ideal spa environment with soft music, white fluffy towels, no phones, or disturbances, fresh flowers and herbs, comfortable chairs and places to relax and chat quietly.

Before using the recipes shown in the following pages,
please make sure to test them on a tiny patch of skin on
your forearm to ensure there are no allergic reactions.

You may not want to mix your chemical facial products with these natural
remedies; they oftentimes don't combine well if you have sensitive skin.

Spa Teas

Chilled Cucumber, Mint and Raspberry Green tea

Delicious during the hot summer months for your spa parties; perfect for reducing aging signs and improving skin tone.

Ingredients
4 cups of hot water
4 tsp of green tea or 4 green tea bags.
1 whole cucumber, sliced
2-3 sprigs of fresh mint
Ice cubes
Raspberries

Directions
1. In a large Pyrex glass jug, add the green tea and pour in the hot boiled water.
2. Allow to steep for 4 minutes; the longer you steep, the stronger the flavor. You may wish to add a small amount of sugar at this point, or honey to sweeten if you are new to green tea.
3. Strain the tea into another glass jug, and refrigerate until cold.
4. Once chilled, add the sliced cucumber, mint, and stir.
5. Fill a pretty jug with ice, and pour in the tea.
6. Lastly, add four raspberries per person to the jug, gently stirring, and serve with a sprig of mint and a slice of cucumber on the side of the jug to decorate.

Experiment with this tea since you may wish to add some lemon slices, more honey (while the tea is hot so that the honey melts), or add other fruits like antioxidant-rich blueberries.

⊂ ⊃ The Sparkling Pomegranate Reviver ⊂ ⊃

For radiant skin, serve this refreshing drink either warm in the winter or on ice in the summer. The potent antioxidants found in pomegranate and white tea combine to bring you clear radiant skin. Since white tea is less caffeinated than green tea, you may find you can drink more of it during the day and avoid caffeine highs.

Ingredients
2 cups of hot water
4 tsp of white tea
2 cups of pomegranate juice
Fresh pomegranate seeds
Ice cubes
2 sliced fresh oranges

Directions
1. In a large Pyrex jug, pour the slightly cooled boiled water over the white tea. Allow to steep for 5-6 minutes. Strain the tea and refrigerate until cold.
2. Add the pomegranate seeds, juice and fresh orange slices to the tea, mixing well.
3. Fill a pretty glass jug with ice, and pour in the tea blend, serving with orange peel twists in each glass.

Beauty Treatments

Facial Saunas

Over a bowl of steaming, but not boiling water, add:

Ingredients

2 drops of Bulgarian rose essential oil –to hydrate dry/mature skin

or

2 drops of lavandula angustifolia essential oil – to calm and soothe

or

2 drops of lemon - to balance oily skin

Directions

Place a towel over your head and bowl, and steam for up to 5 minutes, remembering to come up for air. Then rinse with very cold water.

Tea to Drink: Green tea with a slice of lemon.

Facial Splashes

For an uplifting refreshing facial splash, choose one of the following essential oils and add two drops:

Ingredients

Lavender – to calm and reduce redness.

Rose – to smooth.

Lemon – to tone and tighten.

Tea Tree – to clear and balance oily skin.

Problem Skin

- *For eczema, sunburn and rashes,* soak a cotton ball in cold *rooibos* tea and apply to the affected area to help reduce inflammation. In addition, research shows that 3 cups of *oolong* tea daily may improve eczema.
- *For acne and rosacea,* 4 fl oz of cooled lavender tea with 30 drops of lavender essential oil applied daily, using a spray or a cotton tip to the affected area. This will help reduce redness.
- *For boils,* apply a warm compress to the affected area, and then apply one drop of lavender essential oil to a cotton tip and place directly on the boil every hour. This should bring the boil to a head. Once the pus has been removed, apply tea tree essential oil to the area to help dry and heal. Once the boil has started to heal, use lavender directly on the area for a few days to prevent scarring.
- *For cold sores,* soak a cotton tip in 1 teaspoon of lemon balm tea mixed with a drop of melissa essential oil; apply to the affected area 4 times a day.

Anti-Aging Skin Balancing Green Tea Tonics

Drinking green tea has been shown to slow down the signs of aging as well as applying it to your skin. Hibiscus tea and pomegranate tea will also benefit your skin; so whether you are drinking them iced or hot, make sure you add these refreshing teas to your skin care regime.

Lemon Green Tea Tonic for Oily Skin

Ingredients

4 fl oz blue glass bottle/100 ml with spray plus one 1 fl oz glass bottle with spray top

4 tsp of loose green tea or 2 tea bags with ½ cup of boiling water

1 tablespoon of witch hazel

40 drops of lemon essential oil

10 drops of lavender angustifolia essential oil

Directions

1. In a Pyrex jug, pour the water over the loose green tea and steep until completely cold. Avoid adding essential oils to hot water, or you will lose some of their therapeutic value through the steam.

2. Strain the tea and pour into the large bottle.

3. Add the witch hazel and then the essential oils, shaking the bottle as you go. Give the bottle a good final shake for about 20 seconds, label and then refrigerate for a day.

4. Decant some of the liquid into the smaller bottle to keep in your bag for a refreshing tonic. Keep the tonic refrigerated at all times.

5. Use your lemon tonic after cleansing. Use daily but avoid the sun.

Tea to Drink: Green or white tea.

Lemon Mint Green Tea Tonic - To Minimize Pores

Ingredients

4 fl oz blue glass bottle/100 ml with spray plus one 1 fl oz
   glass bottle with spray top
3 tsp of loose dried peppermint tea, or one tea bag, with ½
   cup of boiling water
3 tablespoons of witch hazel
40 drops of lemon essential oil
10 drops of peppermint essential oil

Directions

1. In a Pyrex, jug pour the water over the tea and steep until
   completely cold. Avoid adding essential oils to hot water,
   or you will lose some of their therapeutic value through
   the steam.
2. Strain the tea and pour into the large bottle.
3. Add the witch hazel, then the essential oils, shaking the
   bottle as you go. Give the bottle a good final shake for
   about 20 seconds, label and then refrigerate for a day.
4. Decant some of the liquid into the smaller bottle to keep
   in your bag for a refreshing tonic. Keep the tonic refrigerated at all times.
5. Use your lemon and mint tonic at night, and in the morning, after cleansing, to tone and close pores. Take your
   small bottle of tonic to work to spritz and refresh your
   skin. Avoid using during the day if you are out in the sun.

*Note: You can replace the dried tea leaves with a tablespoon of fresh
peppermint leaves from the garden, to add extra zing.*

Tea to Drink: Peppermint with a slice of lemon.

Rose Green Tea Tonic -
For Dry, Sensitive or Sunburned Skin

Ingredients

4 fl oz blue glass bottle/100 ml with spray plus one 1 fl oz
   glass bottle with spray cap.

3 tsp of loose green tea with ½ cup of boiling water

1 tsp. of loose rose bud tea

25 drops of Bulgarian rose essential oil

25 drops of lavender angustifolia essential oil

Directions

1. In a Pyrex jug, pour the water over the tea and steep until
   completely cold. Avoid adding essential oils to hot water,
   or you will lose some of their therapeutic value through
   the steam.

2. Strain the tea and pour into the large bottle.

3. Add the essential oils, shaking the bottle as you go. Give
   the bottle a good final shake for about 20 seconds, label
   and then refrigerate for a day.

4. Decant some of the liquid into the smaller bottle to keep
   in your bag for a refreshing tonic. Keep the tonic refrigerated at all times.

5. Use your rose tonic in the morning, daytime, and evening to restore and hydrate. Use the small bottle of tonic
   to carry with you.

Tea to Drink: Loose green tea with rose buds or loose
dried lavender. Add honey to sweeten.

Lavender Green Tea Tonic - To Tone and Cool Normal Skin

Ingredients

4 fl oz blue glass bottle/100 ml with spray plus one 1 fl oz
  glass bottle with spray cap.
3 tsp of loose green tea with ½ cup of boiling water
1 tsp of loose lavender tea (no black tea leaves)
30 drops of lavender angustifolia essential oil

Directions

1. In a Pyrex jug, pour the hot water over the green and rose
    tea; steep until completely cooled down.
2. Strain the tea and pour into the large bottle.
3. Add the essential oils gradually, shaking the bottle as you
    go.
4. Give the bottle a good final shake for about 20 seconds,
    label and then refrigerate for a day. Decant some of the
    liquid into the smaller bottle to keep in your handbag for
    a refreshing tonic. Keep the tonic refrigerated at all times.
5. Use your lavender tonic in the morning, daytime and eve-
    ning to cool inflamed skin; maintain normal skin tone,
    and a healthy glow.

⸎ Tea to Drink: Loose green tea, loose dried lavender. Add
honey to sweeten.

( ) Hydrating Rose Mask ( )

To make a rejuvenating facial mask, mix time-tested ingredients from ancient civilizations for a glowing complexion.

Ingredients
A clean jar
2 tablespoons of liquid honey
2 tsp of jojoba oil
5 drops of Bulgarian rose essential oil

Directions
Mix all ingredients well and massage over clean skin. Relax for 15 minutes, allowing the mask to absorb into the skin. Rinse and then spray with the rose green tea tonic. See overleaf.

Tea to Drink: If its summer, use the sparking pomegranate reviver; if its winter, a warm green or white tea.

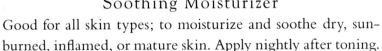

Rose and Lavender
Soothing Moisturizer

Good for all skin types; to moisturize and soothe dry, sun-burned, inflamed, or mature skin. Apply nightly after toning.

Ingredients

2 fl oz glass bottle with cap

2 fl oz of jojoba oil

4 tea rosebuds

3 drops of geranium rose essential oil

Directions

Pour the oil into the bottle, then insert 4 dried rosebuds into the bottle, and add the geranium rose essential oil. Leave for 2-3 days in a cool dark place. Do not refrigerate.Shake well before applying as a nighttime nourishing oil treatment. *Jojoba will not clog the pores on your skin. The oil mimics the skin's natural sebum.*

Tea to Drink: Chamomile tea to relax.

Tea Baths

• *To relax your mind and body*

Stir 1 tablespoon of dried lavender with 8 drops of lavender essential oil. Fill a small muslin bag with the mix and tie with a pretty ribbon. When you run your bath, tie the bag under the tap and allow the water to run through the bag, or let the bag float in the water as you are filling the bath. Tie the bag tightly so it doesn't split. Relax and soak.

• *To relax your muscles at the end of a very long day*

Add 2 tablespoons of Epsom salts to your bath to relax your muscles, and then take two ginger tea bags, apply 3 drops of ginger essential oil to each bag and once the bath is filled, float the bags in the bathwater. Relax and enjoy.

• *For a romantic night*

Stir 1 tablespoon of dried rose buds with 9 drops of Bulgarian rose essential oil. Fill a small muslin bag with the mix and tie with a pretty ribbon. When you run your bath, let the bag float in the water. Before your partner arrives, sprinkle a few rose petals onto the water; not too many as they can get soggy and stick to the skin - not so romantic. Light some candles, pop a bottle of bubbly, or serve a tea cocktail, and voila!

> • *To awaken and invigorate yours senses at the beginning of the day* Take a peppermint tea bag and add 3 drops of peppermint essential oil to the bag. Place it in the bath.

Foot Soaks : Any of these baths can be created as luxurious foot soaks by adding the teas and oils to a large bowl of warm water, and soaking your feet for 10 minutes. These foot soaks are ideal for older people, or those physically unable to take baths. Foot soaks are a delightful experience relaxing the whole body.

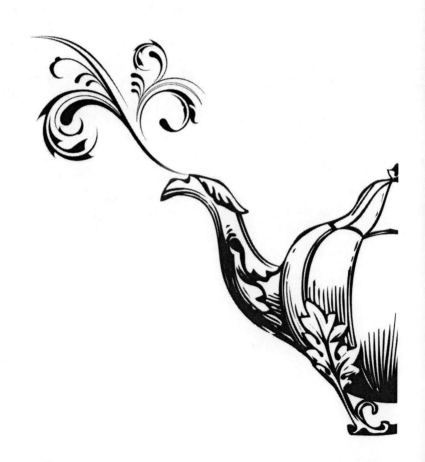

Tea Remedies and Aromatic Elixirs
For Weight Loss

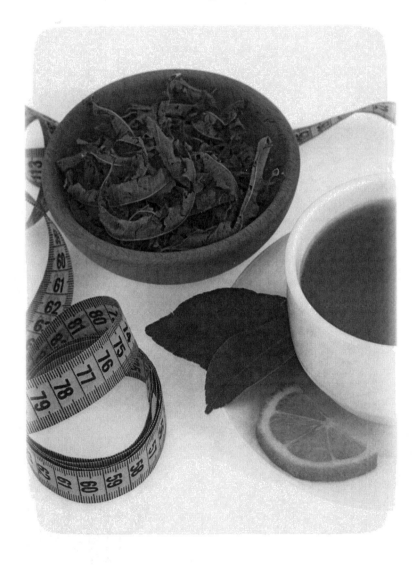

"You must act as if it is impossible to fail."
- Ashanti Proverb

Weight Loss with Tea

"If you don't need a pill to get fat,
why would you need one to get unfat?"
- Unknown

Teas are still being researched for their effectiveness in weight loss. The Chinese have long believed that *oolong* tea is beneficial in reducing and keeping weight off. It can also help control fat metabolism; drinking it twice a day helps to burn calories.

Weight loss pills often contain ingredients that can create additional health problems. Some, for example, have high percentages of caffeine, to speed up the metabolism. Using natural ingredients like tea may help support you in your weight loss program, and will be beneficial to your health.

Weight Loss Teas

☞ Black tea – contains flavonoids that keep fat off and block starches from being absorbed into the body, thereby stopping the buildup of belly fat before it even gets the chance to start.

꒐ *Oolong* tea– helps the body burn a higher number of calories faster, and ramps up your metabolism to continue burning fat for two hours after drinking it. It can maintain weight loss.

꒐ Green tea – helps the body to lose moderate body weight but may not help keep fat off long-term.

꒐ *Matcha* powdered green tea – helps the body to increase thermogenesis (burn calories) by 35–43 percent compared to the average daily burn, which is 8–10 percent.

꒐ Yerba Mate Tea – can subdue your cravings, ensuring you avoid empty calories. It doesn't lead to caffeine crashes, and will give you energy for about four hours. However, studies show that you should drink this tea in moderation; if taken in large quantities (1 litre per day) it may cause cancer

Adding spices to your tea to speed up fat metabolism

Research shows that using spices may speed up your metabolism to help you lose weight. However, as you know, address your eating habits, follow a low-fat diet and take up regular exercise if you want to lose weight and keep it off.

You can add any one of the spices shown to the tea of your choice, as part of your weight loss regime, however, check with your health care provider beforehand. *It is advisable to eat something light before drinking your spiced tea to avoid nausea.*

Cayenne pepper can stimulate the metabolism by about 20 percent to burn calories, and may cause intense sweating. It also has a high content of vitamins, especially vitamin E. Use a quarter teaspoon or less, in your tea.

Cinnamon causes weight loss by heating up the body and stabilizing blood sugar by making cells more responsive to insulin. The antioxidant levels found in cinnamon are highly potent and much higher than well-known sources such as dried blueberries. Cinnamon may also prevent unwanted blood clotting and candida. Use a quarter teaspoon or less of cinnamon in your tea.

Cumin seeds are high in potassium, protein, iron, thiamine, and potent antioxidants, which enhance the spice's ability to detoxify the liver and stimulate weight loss. Grind 2–3 seeds into powder and add to your tea.

Mustard is a useful heat-raising weight loss herb that boosts the metabolic rate by almost 25 percent. High in vitamins, minerals, and other nutrients, mustard is best bought as a powder. As a weight-loss agent, prepared mustard is less effective than the powdered form. Add a quarter teaspoon or less to your tea.

Garlic cleans and detoxifies the body as well as stabilizes blood sugar. It fights cancer and heart disease; lowers blood pressure, cholesterol; and is both antibiotic and anti-fungal. Avoid garlic if you are taking an anticoagulant medicine or have a bleeding disorder. Use one sliver of fresh garlic and add 8 fl oz of hot water to make garlic tea.

Directions for adding a weight-reducing spice to your tea:

Take one teaspoon of loose black, green or *oolong* tea; add ¼ teaspoon or less (depending on your taste) of your chosen spice; stir in with the tea; add 8 fl oz of hot water; allow to steep for 3–4 minutes then strain. You may need to add a tiny amount of honey or lemon to taste. The less time you brew the tea, the lighter the taste will be.

Tea Remedies and Aromatic Elixirs
Stress Busters

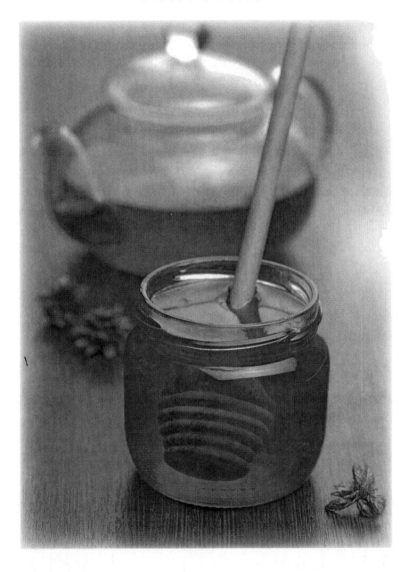

"I don't feel much like Pooh today," said Pooh. "There, there,"
said Piglet, "I'll bring you some tea and honey until you do."
-Winnie the Pooh

Calm and Relax

This remedy is ideal for the evening or bedtime.

Tea Remedy

Ingredients: 1 tsp of chamomile and or lavender tea, loose or in bag, honey to taste.

Directions: Pour 8 fl oz hot water over 1 tsp of loose tea and allow to steep for 3 minutes, or longer, depending on your taste. Strain and add honey.

Essential Oil Elixir

Roman chamomile and Lavender angustifolia.

Ingredients for a Massage/Bath Blend
1 tsp of sweet almond oil
1 drop of chamomile roman
3 drops of lavender angustifolia

Directions
Run your bath and mix up your blend; pour into the bath and soak for 10 minutes. Towel dry and go straight to bed with your hot tea (see above). If a bath is not possible, try a foot bath by filling a large bowl with warm water and adding the oils to the water. Soak your feet for 10 minutes.

For daytime relaxation, use the same essential oil remedy and apply to your wrists, behind your knees, chest and earlobes throughout the day. Chamomile tea can make you sleepy so don't drive after drinking it.

⟨ ⟩ Sleep ⟨ ⟩

These remedies are ideal for those having trouble falling asleep.
As always, it is best to avoid caffeine during the day and relax
with some gentle exercise like *Qi Gong* or yoga in the evening.
Avoid watching TV in bed as it can overstimulate the brain.

⅔ Tea Remedy

Ingredients: 1 tsp of lavender flowers and 1 tsp of lemon balm
tea, either fresh or dried.

Directions: Pour 8 fl oz hot water over the tea and allow to steep
for 3 minutes or longer depending on your taste. Add honey if
needed. Drink in the evening, and upon retiring to bed.

⁏ Essential Oil Elixir

Roman Chamomile, Lavender angustifolia, Jasmine   —

Ingredients for a Room Spray
30 ml blue glass bottle with spray top filled with distilled water
1 drop roman chamomile
3 drops jasmine
4 drops lavender

Directions
Add the oils to the water in the glass bottle, shake well, and
spray liberally around your head, inhaling deeply during the
day to relax. At night, use the same spray and, but also add 1
drop of jasmine, 3 drops of lavender to 1 tsp of sweet almond
oil, and pour this mix in the bath. Relax in bed afterwards
with the hot tea as shown above.

Before retiring, apply one drop of lavender under your nose
and massage each outer ear with lavender. Put 2-3 drops on
your pillow at night as this may also improve sleep.

Tension Headaches

Feeling overwhelmed at work or with family? Spending too long at the computer? Tension in the shoulders can spread into the neck and create headaches. There are different types of headaches that vary in intensity. You will also find recipes for sinus and migraine headaches later in the book.

Tea Remedy

Ingredients: 1 tsp green tea with 1 drop of lavender essential oil, or *rooibus* tea

Directions: Add 1 drop of lavender oil to a teaspoon of loose green tea, then pour 16 fl oz of hot water over the tea, and allow to steep for 2 minutes. Add honey.

For *rooibos* tea, add 8 fl oz of hot water to 1 tsp of tea and allow to steep for 3 minutes. Strain and add honey.

Essential Oil Elixir

Lavender angustifolia, Geranium, Bergamot

Ingredients for a Massage/Bath Blend
1 fl oz/30 ml blue glass bottle with cap filled with sweet
   almond oil
6 drops lavender angustifolia
3 drops geranium
6 drops bergamot

Directions
Add the essential oils to the sweet almond oil in the glass bottle, shake well, and massage your neck and shoulders hourly with the blend. Also add 1 cap to the bath at night, or use after showering.

Room Diffuser: Add up to 6 drops of lavender and 3 drops of geranium to your candle burner or electric room diffuser to help you stay relaxed.

⸎ ⸎ Muscular Pain ⸎ ⸎

For aches and pains that come from sitting for too long at
your desk, in the car, or after an injury.

⸎ Tea Remedy

Ingredients: Fresh ginger root or *rooibos* tea

Directions: Place 4 slices of fresh ginger in the teapot with 8
fl oz of hot water, and steep for 10 minutes. You can either
make *rooibos* separately or add a slice of fresh ginger or a tiny
dash of ginger powder to 1 tsp of the loose tea, and then
add the 8 fl oz of boiling water. Drink either tea regularly
throughout the day.

⸎ Essential Oil Elixir

Lavender angustifolia, Rosemary (avoid with high blood
pressure), Marjoram.

Ingredients for a Massage/Bath Blend
1 fl oz/30 ml blue glass bottle with cap filled with sweet
    almond oil
6 drops lavandula angustifolia
5 drops rosemary
3 drops marjoram

Directions
Add the essential oils to the sweet almond oil in the glass
bottle, shake well, and after showering, massage your whole
body and your armpits with the oil. At night, add 2 tablespoons of Epsom salts and 2 caps of oil to the bath just before
getting in, and soak for 10 minutes.

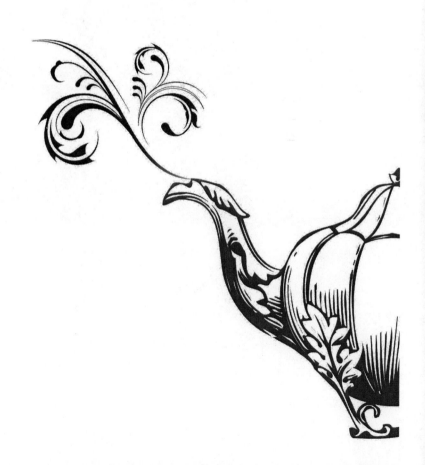

Tea Remedies and Aromatic Elxirs
For Good Health and
Your Immune System

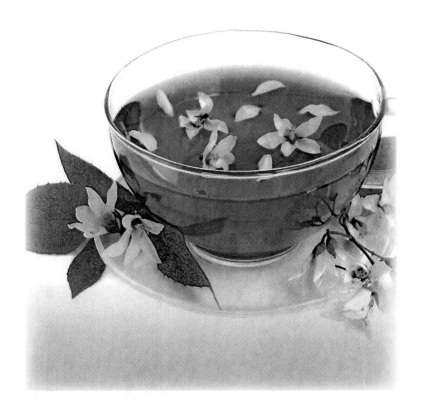

*"The art of medicine consists of amusing
the patient while nature cures the disease."*
-Voltaire

⟨ ⟩ Your Immune System ⟨ ⟩

If you find yourself continually catching flu, colds, sinus infections or allergies of all kinds, you might want to consider building up your immune system with the help of your health care provider.

℘ Tea Remedy

Ingredients: Echinacea, *oolong,* green tea, powdered green *matcha,* pomegranate, white tea

Directions: Choose one of the above teas to benefit your immune system; their brewing methods can be found earlier on in the book. Drink 2-3 cups daily as a preventative measure.

⚛ Essential Oil Elixir

Lavender angustifolia, Eucalyptus globulus, Rosemary cineol, Tea Tree, Oregano, Thyme

Ingredients for a Room/Body Spray:
2 fl oz/50 ml blue glass bottle with spray top filled with
    distilled water
5 drops lavandula angustifolia
5 drops rosemary cineol
10 drops tea tree
5 drops eucalyptus

Directions
Add the essential oils to the sprayer bottle filled with water, shake and use around your home and office as a preventative measure during the cold and flu season. Spray your children's hands with it when they come home from school. Spray tissues with the mix and place in a ziplock bag to be used during the day as hand wipes. Also use the blend in a room diffuser at home or the office.

ꜥ ꜣ For a Cold/Flu ꜥ ꜣ

ꝫ Tea Remedy

Three garlic cloves, or 1 tsp echinacea loose tea, or 4 slices of ginger and fresh lemon juice

Directions: Choose from the selection of remedies above and then either: take 1 tsp of loose echinacea tea and add 8 fl oz of boiling water, drink 2 cups daily. Or, chop 3 garlic cloves and infuse in 2 cups of boiling water for 3 minutes, strain and add half a lemon and honey to taste. Or, slice 4 pieces of ginger instead of the garlic and add lemon and honey after straining. Drink 2-3 cups daily. *If you are taking an anticoagulant or have a bleeding disorder check with your MD before using garlic.*

ꝯ Essential Oil Elixir

Eucalyptus globulus, Ginger, Peppermint (avoid with high blood pressure), Tea Tree.

Ingredients for a Massage/Bath Blend
1 fl oz/30 ml blue glass bottle with screw cap filled with
　　sweet almond oil
7 drops of peppermint
5 drops of eucalyptus
3 drops of tea tree

Directions
Add the essential oils to the bottle filled with sweet almond oil, shake and use one capful for a relaxing bath combined with 3 tablespoons Epsom salts. Go straight to bed to stay warm, with your ginger or garlic tea. Do not come out until well!

Continued on next page

For congestion: Fill the sink in your bathroom with hot water, not boiling. Add half a capful of oil. With a towel over your head; inhale the aromatic steam for 5 minutes, remembering to come up for air during this time. Repeat two to three times a day. Avoid this method if you have asthma.

Sinus Infections/Headaches

Tea Remedy
Ingredients: Peppermint loose leaf, or a peppermint tea bag.

Directions: Using a tablespoon of fresh peppermint or 1 tsp of dried peppermint, add 1 drop of peppermint oil, mix well and then add 8 fl oz of boiling water. Allow to steep for 3-4 minutes or longer. Take the lid off the pot and inhale deeply. Peppermint is known to help clear sinuses. The heat and aroma of the tea may help alleviate sinus pressure when taken 2-3 times a day.

Essential Oil Elixir
Peppermint and Tea Tree

Ingredients for a Spray
1 fl oz/30 ml blue glass bottle with spray top filled with previously boiled distilled water
2 drops peppermint
3 drops tea tree

Directions
Fill the bottle with the water and add the essential oils. Shake well.

Continued on next page

You can either spray a small amount onto a cotton tip, and gently wipe just inside the nostrils, or gently spray into the opening of each nostril. Avoid spraying up into the nose.

Using a Neti pot filled with cooled boiled water, pour 5 drops of the mixed blend into the pot and proceed to use as directed to cleanse the sinuses. If you prefer a stronger solution, add 1 drop of tea tree only – without the other oils – to the water in the Neti pot.

To steam the sinuses, add 1 drop of tea tree and 1 drop of peppermint directly into the sink filled with hot but not boiling water. If the sinus infection persists, then add 1 drop of oregano to the other oils. Steam for up to 5 minutes, coming up for air, twice daily.

Avoid steam inhalation if you have asthma.

⟨ ⟩ For Air Travel ⟨ ⟩

⟩ Tea Remedy

Peppermint and green teabags. The hostesses bring hot water for tea so you can use your own teabags. Drink peppermint for your sinuses and green tea for your immune system.

Directions for a Travel Size Body Spray Elixir:
Use the same essential oils for the immune spray in a 1 fl oz sprayer bottle for the plane. This spray can be used to protect you from bacteria, viruses and help keep your sinuses clear. Spray on your seat, and on your hands. You can also gently mist it around you when in the bathroom, so you don't disturb anyone with the fragrance. I even put some inside my nostrils to counteract bacteria/germs.

In addition, carry a small 10 ml bottle of tea tree with you, and if you prefer something stronger, you can use this as a hand sanitizer and also place a drop inside each nostril to prevent germs.

Tea Remedies and Aromatic Elxirs
For Your Heart

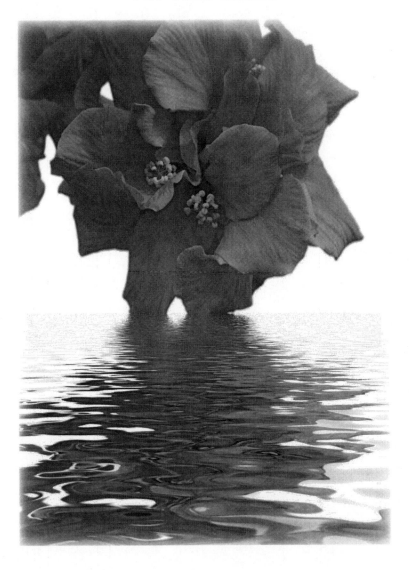

"There are always flowers for those who want to see them."
-Henri Matisse

⟨ ⟩ High Blood Pressure ⟨ ⟩

There are of course many reasons for high blood pressure. Obesity, stress, lack of exercise, anger, hormones, heart complications, and poor kidney function may be just some of the contributing factors. The intention is to treat the whole body with these remedies with agreement from your health care provider.

Choosing some teas from the Stress Busting chapter and taking time to relax, exercise and eating consciously will also help. Using essential oils to help calm the nervous system may also aid in reducing your blood pressure.

❧ Tea Remedy

Ingredients: Hibiscus tea, avoiding all other teas even with lower caffeine content i.e. green and white.

Directions: For ease you can purchase dried hibiscus flowers or tea bags. Pour boiling water over 2 tsps of hibiscus flowers and allow to infuse for 3–4 minutes. Drink up to 3 cups daily for 6 weeks.

❦ Essential Oil Elixir

Lavender angustifolia, *ylang ylang*

Directions for a Massage/Bath Blend
2 fl oz/50 ml blue glass bottle with cap filled with sweet almond oil
15 drops lavandula angustifolia
10 drops *ylang ylang*

Continued on next page

Directions
Add the essential oils to the bottle filled with oil; shake and use a capful in the bath nightly. Or, after showering, massage the chest and under the armpits for extra absorption twice daily.

At night, massage the soles of your feet with the oil before getting into bed and massage around the earlobes before sleep. You can also add 2-3 drops of lavender to your pillow.

Low Blood Pressure

Just as high blood pressure can stress the body, so can low blood pressure, which can cause bouts of dizziness, weakness and fatigue. Avoid lavender essential oil as it may lower your blood pressure even further.

Tea Remedy

Ingredients: Green, white, peppermint or black tea.

Directions: Take 1 tsp of one of the above loose teas and add 8 fl oz of boiling water. Allow to steep for 4 minutes or longer. The longer you steep the tea, the higher the caffeine content, thereby raising blood pressure. For peppermint tea, add 1 drop of peppermint essential oil to the tea before adding the hot water. Drink 2-3 cups daily.

Essential Oil Elixir
Peppermint, Rosemary, Black Pepper

Directions for a Massage/Bath Blend
2 fl oz/50 ml blue glass bottle with cap filled with sweet almond oil
10 drops peppermint
8 drops rosemary
1 drop black pepper

Continued on next page

Directions
Add the essential oils to the bottle filled with oil, shake and use a capful in the bath in the morning. Or after showering, massage the chest and under the armpits for extra absorption. Use throughout the day on your pulse points and ear lobes. You can also make the same blend into a 2 fl oz spray but using distilled water instead of sweet almond oil. Use the spray to uplift and stimulate your senses up until about 5 pm. Avoid using the oils until the next morning as, like caffeine, the oils may keep you awake at night!

Tea for reducing the risk of heart attacks
Black tea- has proven to be effective in lowering the risk of heart attacks. People who have been drinking black tea for at least a year are less likely to die from a heart attack.

Tea for stroke prevention
Green tea – research indicates that drinking three cups of green tea daily lowers the risk of having a stroke; compared to drinking one cup daily or none. Women seemed to benefit more than men.

Tea Remedies and Aromatic Elxirs
For Women's Health

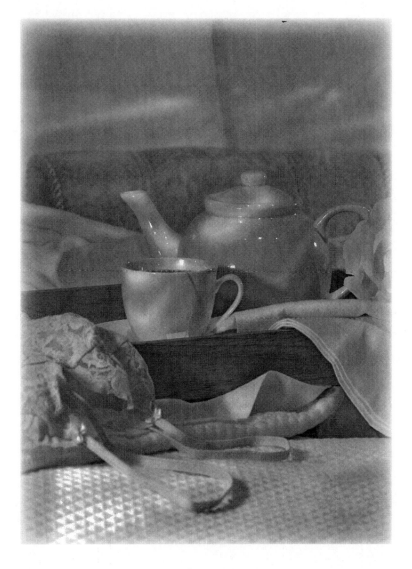

"Women are like teabags, they don't know how strong
they are until they get into hot water."
- Eleanor Roosevelt

⸨ ⸩ Regulate ⸨ ⸩

For irregular menstrual cycles, painful periods, and PMS symptoms, including excessive bleeding and cramps, raspberry leaf tea, combined with a healthy diet and exercise may help to bring balance and regularity.

❧ Tea Remedy

Ingredients: Raspberry leaf tea

Directions: Place 1 tsp of loose tea in the teapot with 8 fl oz of hot water, and allow to steep for 10 minutes. Drink 2 cups daily.

❦ Essential Oil Elixir

Clary Sage, Geranium, Lavender angustifolia, Nutmeg

Directions for a Massage/Bath Blend
1 fl oz/30 ml blue glass bottle with cap filled with sweet
   almond oil
2 drops lavandula angustifolia
7 drops clary sage
4 drops geranium
2 drops nutmeg

Directions
Add the essential oils to the sweet almond oil in the glass bottle, shake well, and after showering massage your whole body, your armpits, and your belly with the oil. At night, add 1 cap of the oil to the bath just before getting in and soak for 10 minutes.

⟨ ⟩ Easing Menopause ⟨ ⟩

Looking at the word menopause, you might see the phrase "putting men on pause" as an alternative meaning for this time in your life that can be uncomfortable, frustrating, and disorienting. On an emotional level, menopause can be seen as a time to become more connected with who you are. It could be a time to reveal the real you and see what you are prepared to deal with and what you aren't; what you want from life and what you don't. With this upheaval in your hormones, you'll probably find yourself more open to speaking the truth, and be less willing to stand for nonsense! Your body is taking you into a new way of being, and a new phase of your life.

The following remedies may support you during this transitional process of hot flashes and dramatic mood swings.

ᕗ Tea Remedy

Ingredients: Honey Bush Tea, raspberry Leaf tea, red clover tea – reported to ease hot flashes and increase bone density.

Directions: Place 1 tsp of either of the above loose teas in the teapot with 8 fl oz of hot water and allow to steep for 10 minutes. Drink 2 cups daily.

⚝ Essential Oil Elixir

Clary Sage, Geranium, Lavender angustifolia, Lemon

Directions for a Massage/Bath Blend
1 fl oz/30 ml blue glass bottle with cap filled with sweet
    almond oil and 1 capsule of evening primrose oil
2 drops lavandula angustifolia
4 drops clary Sage
3 drops geranium
 6 drops lemon   *Continued on next page*

Add the essential oils to the sweet almond oil in the glass bottle, shake well. After showering, massage your whole body and your armpits with the oil. At night, add 1 cap of the oil to the bath just before getting in, and soak for 10 minutes. Do this daily.

For night sweats, keep a bottle of lemon and lavender spray by your bed. Fill a 100 ml bottle with water and add 40 drops of lavender and 25 drops of lemon to use over your body as needed.

⟨ ⟩ Kidneys & Bladder ⟨ ⟩

Keeping the kidneys flushed and free from stones and infection can be done with drinking 1 liter of water a day. Included in that fluid intake can be the consumption of black tea, which is known to reduce the risk of kidney stones. *Oolong* tea may also eliminate toxins through the kidneys, and can be a mild diuretic. Always check with your health provider.

❧ Tea Remedy for the Kidneys

Ingredients: Black tea, *oolong* tea, green tea, *rooibos*

Directions: Choose one of the above teas according to your preference, and add 1 tsp to the teapot with 8 fl oz of hot water and allow to steep for 3-4 minutes. Drink 2 cups daily.

❧ Essential Oil Elixir

Juniper, Rosemary, Fennel, Lemon

Directions for a Massage/Bath Blend for the kidneys
1 fl oz/30 ml blue glass bottle with cap filled with sweet
   almond oil
4 drops juniper
6 drops rosemary
3 drops fennel
2 drops lemon

Add the essential oils to the sweet almond oil in the glass bottle, shake well. After showering, massage your whole body, including under your armpits and lower back, with the oil. At night, add 1 cap of the oil to the bath just before getting in, and soak for 10 minutes.

Bladder

For regular bladder infections, such as cystitis, which are becoming more resistant to antibiotics, it is important to drink 1 liter of fluid a day, and avoid black tea and coffee. However, in your daily liquid consumption, you could include unsweetened cranberry juice, diluted with purified water, along with cranberry tea.

Tea Remedy for the Bladder

Ingredients: Cranberry tea, green tea, white tea.

Directions: See page 90 for fresh cranberry tea. Alternatively, infuse a cranberry tea bag for 5 minutes, or add a tablespoon of warmed cranberry juice to your green or white tea, adding a slice of lemon and some honey.

Essential Oil Elixir

Rosemary, Oregano, Lavender

Directions for a Massage/Bath Blend for the bladder
1 fl oz/30 ml blue glass bottle with cap filled with sweet
    almond oil
2 drops oregano
8 drops rosemary
2 drops lavender

Add the essential oils to the sweet almond oil in the glass bottle, shake well. After showering, massage your lower hips, pelvis and bladder area with the oil. At night, add 1 cap of the oil to the bath just before getting in, and soak for 10 minutes. Alternatively, you can pour a warm bath just up to your hips, add the oils, and sit soaking for 5 minutes.

Cellulite

Cellulite may be due to water retention, hormonal changes, sluggish lymphatic drainage, lack of exercise, poor diet, and excess weight. Avoid dairy and sugar; eat more raw cabbage (acts as a diuretic); and step up your vitamin and mineral intake with the advice of your health care provider. The following may help manage or improve cellulite.

Tea Remedy

Ingredients: Black tea, *oolong* tea, *pu'erh* tea, green tea.

Directions: Place 1 tsp of either of the above loose teas mixed with a drop of grapefruit or lemon essential oil in a teapot. Add 8 fl oz of hot water, allowing to steep for 3-4 minutes. Drink 2 cups daily.

Essential Oil Elixir

Juniper, Grapefruit, Rosemary, Thyme

Directions for a Massage/Bath Blend
1 fl oz/30 ml blue glass bottle with cap filled with sweet
    almond oil
4 drops juniper
5 drops rosemary
6 drops grapefruit

Directions for an Epsom Salt Bath Blend
16 oz Epsom salts
16 drops of rosemary
30 drops of grapefruit
5 drops of juniper
2 tsps of sweet almond oil

Continued on next page

For the Massage/Bath Blend
Fill your bottle with sweet almond oil and add all essential oils, shake well. This quantity of oil will last only a short while, so I suggest you experiment with this reduced quantity first, and then make a larger quantity for long-term use, enough for a three-month period.

For the Epsom Salt Bath Blend
Add all ingredients into the Epsom salts and stir well; pour the mix into a screw top jar.

1ˢᵗ Step – Breaking down the Cellulite
- Firstly, warm your skin in the shower to open your pores, then massage at least 4 capfuls of the oil blend in upward circular motions all over your body, paying attention to the areas affected with cellulite.
- Spend 5 minutes at the end of your shower, turning the water to as hot as you can bear it without scalding your skin, and directing the shower stream at the cellulite. Then turn the water to as cold as you can handle it, directing the shower stream at the cellulite. Repeat this process for at least 3-5 minutes. The impact of the heat and cold will stimulate the lymphatic system and may help remove toxins.
- Finish with a cold shower, and then use a bristle or loofah brush to briskly brush your body all over in upward movements towards the heart.
- After showering, massage the oil once again over the affected areas while your skin is damp, before towel drying.

2ⁿᵈ Step – Detox Baths
- Twice to three times a week, add 2 tablespoons of Epsom salts to the bath, followed by a capful of massage oil. Making

Continued on next page

sure the water isn't too hot; sit and soak for 10 minutes. Be sure to keep massaging the cellulite while you sit in the bath in order to break down the fat deposits. You can make the Epsom salts ahead of time. Take a cold shower after a bath to continue stimulating the lymphatic system.

3rd Step – Tea
- Enjoy a cup of green or *oolong* tea with half a lemon 2-3 times daily to detox and increase fat metabolism. You can also choose from one of the weight-loss teas.

4th Step – Diet and Exercise
Begin an exercise regime that targets the muscles in the cellutlite-stricken areas by staying off sugar, dairy and any foods that are white! Introduce more vegetable juices, vegetables, chicken, fish, and brown rice into your diet.

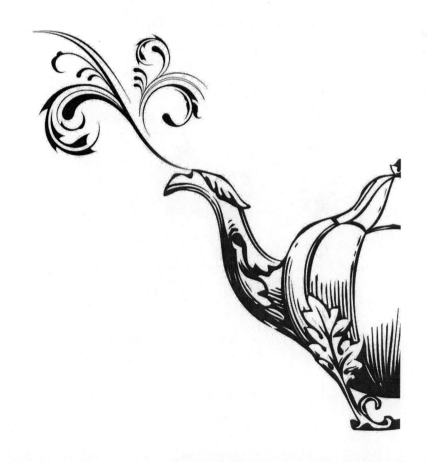

Tea Remedies and Aromatic Elixirs
For Digestion

"Happiness: a good bank account, a good cook, and a good digestion."
- Jean-Jacques Rosseau

⟨ ⟩ Constipation ⟨ ⟩

Dietary changes, inadequate water consumption, and stress can lead to constipation. You can include the remedies from the Stress Buster section with the remedies below. Avoid black tea and coffee since the caffeine can act as a diuretic, leaving you dehydrated. Drink at least 1 liter of water a day, including the teas below.

Tea Remedy
Ingredients: Ginger and fennel,or chai

Directions: Infuse 4 slices of ginger and ¼ tsp of powdered fennel in 8 fl oz of water for 5 minutes, strain and add honey. Then follow the massage as shown below. If you prefer a "warming" blend with more taste, try making a chai tea (see recipe earlier in the book), swapping out dairy for either rice or almond milk.

Essential Oil Elixir
Ginger, Peppermint, Chamomile

Directions for a Massage/Bath Blend
1 fl oz/30 ml blue glass bottle with cap filled with sweet
   almond oil
5 drops ginger
4 drops ginger

Add the essential oils to the sweet almond oil in the glass bottle; shake well. Drink either of the teas above, and then after 20 minutes take a capful of the oil blend and massage your abdomen in a clockwise direction; going as deeply as you can, moving over your hips, your back and down to the buttocks, just above the anus. Repeat the whole process three times a day.

⟨ ⟩ Diarrhea ⟨ ⟩

Avoid dairy, and if the diarrhea is from a bacterial infection, probiotics can often rebalance the intestinal "friendly" bacteria to fight off the invading organisms.

❧ Tea Remedy
Ingredients: Ginger tea, peppermint tea, chamomile tea

Directions: Take 1 tsp of peppermint or chamomile tea and add 8 fl oz of boiled water, still warm not boiling, allow to steep for 3–4 minutes. Strain and add a tsp of honey. For ginger tea, cut 3–4 slices of ginger and allow to infuse in 8 fl oz of boiling water for 5 minutes at least. Then strain and add a tsp of honey.

❦ Essential Oil Elixir
Ginger, Chamomile

Recipe for a Massage/Bath Blend
1 fl oz/30 ml blue glass bottle with cap filled with sweet almond oil. Chose <u>one</u> of the oils from above and add 8–9 drops.

Add one of the essential oils to the sweet almond oil in the glass bottle and shake well. Gently massage the abdomen in a clockwise motion. Finish by placing a warm hot water bottle on the abdomen. If the abdomen is too tender to touch, add 10 drops of oil to a small bowl of hot water (not boiling); soak a thin piece of clean cloth and apply the compress to the abdomen until it cools; then keep reapplying for as long as comfortable.

ᑐ Stomach Acidity ᑕ

Stress may play a role with excess acid and indigestion, revisiting you after each meal. Perhaps your diet or a lack of enzymes could be contributing factors. As you discuss your symptoms with your health provider, you may be encouraged to look at the changes you can make in your lifestyle. Probiotics can often help. Choose calming, gentle foods and avoid caffeine, dairy, sugar, and fried foods.

ᔟ Tea Remedy

Ingredients: Marshmallow tea, chamomile tea, *rooibus* with a sprinkle of fennel, cardamom, coriander. Peppermint tea.

Directions: Take 1 tsp of marshmallow tea and add 8 fl oz of boiling water; allow to steep overnight. Strain and heat gently until warm. Depending on your taste, you may prefer chamomile or *rooibos* tea (with the above spices). Take 1 tsp of either of these teas, add 8 fl oz of boiling water, and steep for 3-4 minutes. Drink any of these teas 2-3 times daily before eating.

If you need fast acid relief, try peppermint tea with honey, and drink after eating. Use the marshmallow tea to soothe your stomach between meals.

ᔟ Essential Oil Elixir

Cardamom, Coriander, Ginger, Peppermint

Directions for a Massage/Bath Blend
1 fl oz/30 ml blue glass bottle with cap filled with sweet almond oil.
5 drops cardamom

Continued on next page

5 drops coriander
6 drops ginger

Add the essential oils to the sweet almond oil in the glass bottle and shake well. Gently massage the upper abdomen in a clockwise motion after each meal.

If stomach acid is intense immediately after meals, blend 5 drops of peppermint in 1 fl oz of sweet almond oil and massage the upper abdomen.

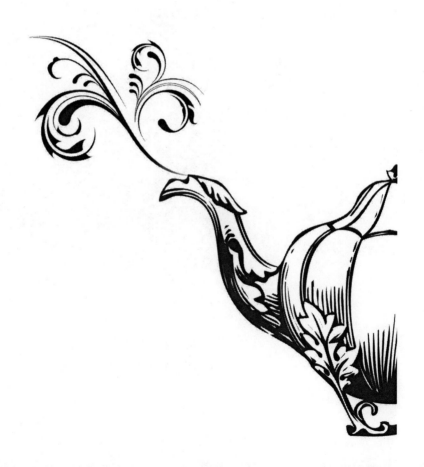

Fresh Aromatic Elxirs
For Your Home and Office

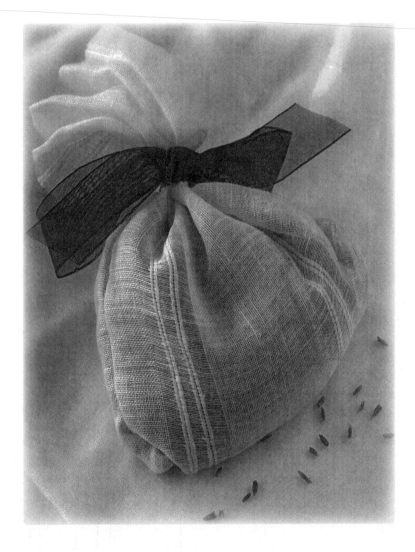

*"You are only here for a short visit: don't hurry, don't worry. And be
sure to smell the flowers along the way."*
-*Walter Hagen*

◌ Ah Now I Remember! – Room Mist ◌
Fresh and clean with a hint of citrus to jolt your memory ...

Recipe
1 tbsp of fresh lemon balm leaves or 1 tsp of dried lemon balm
4 fl oz of boiling water
50 drops of melissa essential oil
5 drops of peppermint essential oil
4 fl oz blue glass bottle with sprayer

Directions: Pour the boiling water onto the lemon balm leaves, allow to cool. Strain and add the melissa essential oil and the peppermint. Pour the liquid into the bottle. Shake well. Label. Spray as required. Keep refrigerated.

◌ Focus – Room and Body Mist ◌
Stimulating and ideal for when you need to meet a deadline, study for an exam, burn the midnight oil, or write a book!

Recipe
1 tbsp of fresh rosemary sprigs or 1 tsp of dried rosemary
4 fl oz of boiling water
50 drops of rosemary essential oil
20 drops of lemon essential oil
4 fl oz blue glass bottle

Directions: Pour the boiling water onto the rosemary; allow to cool. Strain and add the rosemary and lemon essential oils. Shake well. Pour the liquid into the bottle. Label. Spray as required. Makes a good air freshener. Keep refrigerated.

⟨ ⟩ Calm Room Mist ⟨ ⟩

Soothing and relaxing; restores peace and harmony. Ideal for the children's nursery, bedroom, and a good sleep.

Recipe
1 tbsp of dried lavender flowers
1 tsp of dried chamomile flowers
4 fl oz of boiling water
60 drops of lavender angustifolia essential oil
5 drops of roman chamomile essential oil
4 fl oz blue glass bottle

Directions: Pour the boiling water over the lavender and chamomile flowers, allow to cool. Strain and add the lavender and chamomile roman essential oils. Pour into the bottle. Shake well. Label. Spray as required. Keep refrigerated. If no flowers are available, you can add essential oils of lavender and chamomile to distilled water for a good calming spray.

Holiday spice and all things nice!
Enticing Room Mist

A delicious, sweet and spicy fragrance to add to the festive holiday atmosphere. Don't forget to add a drop of pine essential oil to your pine cones before putting them on the tree.

Recipe
3 ginger teabags
4 fl oz of boiling water
1 tsp of orange peel dried or fresh
30 drops of sweet orange essential oil
3 drops of clove essential oil
2 drops of cinnamon essential oil
3 drops of ginger essential oil
2 drops of nutmeg essential oil
4 fl oz blue glass bottle with sprayer

Directions: Pour the boiling water over the ginger teabags and orange peel; leave to cool. Remove the teabags and orange peel after 2 or more hours. Add the essential oils. Pour into the bottle. Shake well. Spray your home before friends and family arrive for celebrating. You can also apply the essential oils above to a piece of tissue and tuck it among your holiday gift wrap to scent it with the fragrances of the season. Keep your gift wrap in a sealed container with the tissue so the fragrance doesn't escape.

Clearing Negative Energy and Energizing – Room Mist

Clear Spray for Natural Positive Energy

When you feel like you have taken on the burdens of the world and you can't seem to shake off that negative energy; or you feel sad for no reason, you may just need to clear and rebalance your energy. I formulated the Clear spray to help you do just that.

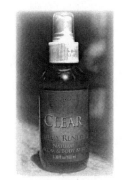

With its refreshing blend of citrus and floral notes, Clear has been used for years by many health practitioners, clients, parents, football teams, children and business people to clear negative emotions, and help focus as well as see things in a more positive light.

You can find the whole range at my website www.aroma1.com.

Potpourri

To maintain a delicious aroma throughout your home, you can become quite creative with dried fruits and teas. Even pouring a ready-made dried fruit tea from the box into a pretty bowl, and adding essential oils of sweet orange, lemon or grapefruit, is easy to do. Citrus oils will evaporate quickly so will need to be topped up every other day.

Recipe for a romantic potpourri
- 10 dried roses
- 4 tbsp of rose bud tea
- 4 tbsp of lavender flower tea
- 2 tbsp of green tea
- 2 tbsp of dried mint leaves
- 30 drops of lavender essential oil
- 10 drops of rose essential oil
- 1 drop of peppermint essential oil

Directions: Combine all of the dried ingredients in a bowl and stir in the essential oils, mixing thoroughly. Pour into a pretty bowl and cover with cling film for a day to allow the oils to absorb, then uncover and enjoy. Stir the potpourri with your hands to release the oils and to scent your skin. Enjoy.

Lavender Bags

Create your own attractive dried lavender bags to hang in your closet to keep the moths away, or slip under your pillow to help you sleep. Earlier in the book, you will find directions for drying lavender in the herbal teas section. There are plenty of suppliers online to purchase pretty small linen bags for your dried lavender, or make your own from left-over remnants of fabric.

'T' Time - Cocktail Hour

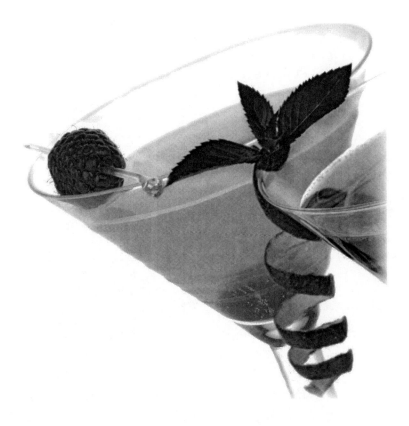

"Everything stops for tea!"

'T' Time!

Looking to jazz up your cocktail hour? Add a splash of healthy tea to a fun mix of non-alcoholic or alcoholic tea cocktails. Not only are they tasty but they're a whole lot better for you.

The following recipes are measured by individual glass servings, so for parties, I suggest you multiply the alcohol quantities shown in each recipe by the number of people attending. To make the tea in bulk, start with two tea bags per 8 fl oz of water and then add or reduce according to taste. You will be able to adjust the sweetness or tartness of each recipe to your liking. Make your cocktail elixir ahead in a glass jug decorated with fruits and mint leaves. Most of all, have fun!

Alcoholic Cocktail "Teanis"

( ) Sparkling "Tea-quila" Sunset ( )

This exhilarating cocktail brings the benefits of black tea's antioxidants with vitamin C in the orange juice, helping your body assimilate the alcohol.

Ingredients
- 1 black tea bag
- 2 fl oz warm water
- ¼ tsp of honey or sugar
- 1 fl oz tequila
- 1 fl oz orange juice
- Prosecco Brut/Sparkling water

Makes one serving.

Directions
1. In a Pyrex jug, pour the warm water over the tea bag and add the sugar or honey. Allow to steep for no longer than 2 minutes as the tea will become bitter and will override the taste of the cocktail. Remove the tea bag and cool the tea in the freezer for 20 minutes.
2. Add ice to your cocktail shaker and pour in the cold tea, tequila, orange juice, and shake vigorously!
3. Pour the blend into your cocktail glass and top up the glass with a splash of Prosecco or sparkling water for a refreshing drink.
4. To decorate, add a fine curl of orange zest.

Cranberry Gin "Marteani"

A light, zingy and tart cocktail ideal for those of you on diets. You can swap out the cranberry tea bag for cranberry juice. However, if you do this, you will be increasing the sugar content.

Ingredients
- 1 cranberry tea bag
- 2 fl oz water
- 1 fl oz gin
- ¼ fl oz lime juice
- 1 fl oz orange juice

Makes one serving.

Directions
1. In a Pyrex jug, pour the warm water over the tea bag and allow to steep for 3 minutes, remove the tea bag and freeze for 20 minutes until cold
2. In a cocktail shaker combine ice, gin, lime and orange juice, tea and shake.
3. Serve in a chilled martini glass with a curl of lime zest.

Brandy Refresher

This cocktail is ideal before or after dinner, but also perfect on its own with appetizers. The green tea addition gives a clean and crisp finish. You can omit the sugar in the green tea if you feel its sweet enough with the ginger ale. In addition, I would suggest making the cocktail and then leaving it to stand for a couple of minutes before drinking it. This way all the ingredients infuse well.

Ingredients
- 2 fl oz warm water
- 1 green tea bag
- ¼ tsp sugar
- 1.25 fl oz brandy
- 2 fl oz ginger ale
- ¼ tsp lemon juice

Makes one serving.

Directions
1. In a Pyrex jug, pour warm water over the tea bag, add the sugar and stir. Allow to steep for only 3 minutes. If you leave it longer, the green tea taste will overwhelm the cocktail.
2. Remove the tea bag and place tea in freezer to cool for 20 minutes.
3. Fill a tumbler with ice. Add the brandy, ginger ale and lemon juice to the tea, and pour over the ice.
4. Decorate with a small curl of lemon zest.
5. Leave to rest for a couple of minutes if you can.

ꙮ Chai Kahlua ꙮ

A comforting and warming drink for the winter months; to be drank on its own with some sweet nibbles, after dinner.

Ingredients
- 3 fl oz of Kahlua
- ½ fl oz of white rum
- ¼ tsp nutmeg
- ¼ tsp cinnamon
- ¼ tsp ginger
- ¼ tsp cardamom
- ½ – 1 tsp of heavy cream

Makes one serving.

Directions
1. Mix the powdered spices in a small bowl.
2. Pour the Kahlua into a glass; add the spices and stir.
3. Add the white rum, stir and add the ice, then stir.
4. Taste and if preferred, add the heavy cream.

Sparkling Hibiscus and Pomegranate Prosecco

A great celebration drink for parties and special occasions, it not only looks pretty in a champagne flute but is full of healthy antioxidants.

Ingredients
- 1 hibiscus tea bag with 2 fl oz of warm water or a hibiscus flower
- 1 fl oz unsweetened pomegranate juice
- 2 fl oz Prosecco Brut or Sweet depending on your preference
- Two champagne glasses
- Mint leaves to decorate

Makes two servings.

Directions
1. In a Pyrex jug, add the water to the tea bag. Allow to steep for 3 minutes and remove the bag. Cool in the freezer for 20 minutes.
2. After the tea is cooled, pour 1 fl oz of tea into each champagne glass; add the pomegranate juice to each glass, and top up with the Prosecco. Decorate with a mint leaf.

Alternatively, if you prefer not to use the hibiscus tea, you can put a clean hibiscus flower at the bottom of the glass and pour the pomegranate juice and Prosecco over it.

⟨ ⟩ Hibiscus Gin and Grapefruit Zinger ⟨ ⟩

This makes a lovely and refreshing afternoon drink, with a little zing to it. Great for afternoon tea parties where guests are sure to admire your recent cocktail creation.

Ingredients
- 1 hibiscus tea bag with 2 fl oz of warm water
- 1 fl oz gin
- 1 fl oz grapefruit juice
- Splash of tonic
- Mint leaves for decoration

Makes one serving.

Directions
1. Pour the warm boiled water over the teabag and allow to steep for three minutes before removing the bag. Cool in the freezer for 20 minutes.
2. Fill a tumbler with ice; pour in the gin and grapefruit juice.
3. Pour in the hibiscus tea, leaving room in the glass for a splash or more of tonic.
4. Serve with a mint leaf.

Non-alcoholic Tea Refreshers

‹ ⟩ Iced Matcha ‹ ⟩

This is a great summer drink for adults and children alike, and a great fun way to celebrate birthdays.

Ingredients
- Prepared green tea *matcha* (see page 65)
- 1 fl oz milk or dairy-free product
- Ice cubes

Directions
1. In a separate glass, whisk the milk or dairy-free product with a bamboo whisk until frothy.
2. Add ice to the glass.
3. Add the warm *matcha*; and sugar or syrup for sweetness.

‹ ⟩ Frozen Matcha Latte ‹ ⟩

A good alternative to a milkshake, packed with nutrients and antioxidants.

Ingredients
- 2 oz sugar or less
- Prepared green tea *matcha*
- 4 fl oz milk or a dairy-free product
- Ice cubes

Directions
1. Prepare your *matcha*, following previous steps shown. (page 65)
2. Add the sugar to your *matcha* mix.
3. In a blender add ice, *matcha* and 4 oz of milk. Blend, pour and enjoy! (Top it with cream for extra indulgence).

Decadent Chocolate Chai

Ingredients
- 1 cup of milk (or dairy alternative)
- ¼ cup of water
- 1 black tea bag (use two if you like your tea very strong)
- 2 tbsp of chocolate syrup
- ½ tsp of pumpkin spice blend (My niece, Olivia, recommends this option) or a combination of cinnamon, ginger and nutmeg – adjust spices to your taste.
- Whipped cream

Directions
1. Boil the milk, spices and water in a pan, stirring occasionally.
2. After the milk boils, return to a low simmer, add the tea bag, and allow to steep for 2 - 3 minutes depending on how strong you like your tea.
3. Remove the tea bag and add the chocolate syrup. Whisk.
4. Pour into a mug and top with whipped cream and shaved milk chocolate, or more chocolate syrup.

Iced Orange Tea

Time to nurture your body with refreshing Vitamin C. This blend is an ideal replacement for your traditional afternoon cup of tea.

Ingredients
- 1 black tea bag
- 2 fl oz warm water
- ½ tsp of honey or sugar
- 2 fl oz orange juice and a slice of orange

Directions
1. In a Pyrex jug pour the warm water over the tea bag and add the sugar or honey. Steep for 2 minutes, no longer as the tea will become bitter. Remove the tea bag and cool the tea in the freezer for 20 minutes.
2. Add ice to your glass, orange juice and a slice of orange, and then pour over your cooled tea.
3. Top up with a splash of sparkling water, if preferred.

⸙ Iced Agua de Jamaica (Hibiscus Tea) ⸙

Give yourself a taste of island life with this delicious blend of flowers, fruits, and spices. Serve at tropical-themed parties; sure to go down well with everyone.

Ingredients
- 1 cup of water
- 1 tsp of sugar or more depending on your taste
- 1 hibiscus tea bag
- 1 slice of fresh ginger
- 1 tsp of lime juice
- Ice and orange slices to garnish
- Splash of tonic to sweeten or sparkling water.

Directions
1. Heat the water and sugar in a pan with the ginger slice.
2. Once the sugar has melted, remove from heat, and add the hibiscus tea bag.
3. Allow to steep for 5 minutes. Remove the tea bag and leave to cool.
4. Remove the ginger. Then add the lime juice, and pour the tea over ice. Garnish with orange slices. You can add sparkling water, tonic or soda for a festive version.

Tea Sweet Treats

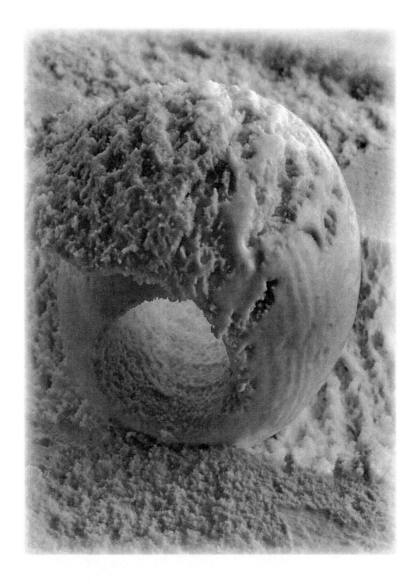

"The word 'Stressed,' spelled backwards, spells desserts. Coincidence?"
-Author unknown

Green Tea Ice Cream

This ice cream takes about 25 minutes to make, and then some time in the ice cream maker to churn and freeze. It is well worth the wait, and will last in the freezer for a couple of days. It has more of a custard feel to it, but if you want something lighter, quicker and egg- free, see Kara's Quick Green Tea Ice Cream recipe over-leaf.

Serve with green tea truffles for true decadence.

Ingredients
¾ cup milk
2 egg yolks
5 tbsp sugar
¾ cup heavy cream, whipped
3 tbsp quality *matcha* green tea powder
Ice cream maker

Makes 4 servings.

Directions
1. Lightly whisk egg yolks in a pan. Add sugar to the eggs while whisking and then gradually pour in the milk.
2. Put the pan on low heat and heat the mixture, stirring continuously, and making sure to scrape the bottom of the pan each time.
3. When the mixture is thickened and lump free, remove the pan from the heat; stir in the green tea powder thoroughly until dissolved. Soak bottom of the pan in ice water to cool the mixture. While it is cooling, whip the cream until thick.
4. Add the cream into the mixture and stir gently.
5. Pour the mixture into an ice cream maker and churn, following the manufacturer's directions.

Kara's Handmade Quick
Green Tea Ice Cream

Made by hand using ziplock bags, this quick and easy recipe is fun to make with the kids. It can be eaten almost immediately - if you like soft ice cream - or put in the freezer for 20 minutes to really firm up. It can also be left for a couple of hours in the freezer before eating. Kara is 12, and makes this for her family.

Ingredients
¾ cup of heavy cream
¼ cup 2 percent milk
3 tbsp sugar
1 tbsp *matcha* quality green tea powder (if you use a sweet-
　　ened green tea powder, use only
　　2 ½ tbsp of sugar)
8 tbsp salt with 5 cups of ice
1 strong plastic gallon bag with zipper and 1 strong quart
　　bag with zipper.

Makes 4 servings.

Directions
1.　Pour all ingredients - minus the salt and ice - into a large
　　Pyrex jug. Mix well.
2.　Place the ice and salt in the large gallon bag.
3.　Taking the smaller quart bag, pour the icecream mix in
　　the jug into the bag, push the air out and seal well. Place
　　this bag inside the larger bag with the ice and salt. Push
　　the air out and seal the larger bag well. Continued on next page

4. Cover the ziplock bag with a hand towel or something to protect your hands from the cold.

5. Shake the bag vigorously in all directions for 5 minutes over the sink. Check on the smaller bag inside containing the ice cream, which will become smooth and thick. Kara recommends shaking the bag for 5 minutes at least.

6. Remove the smaller bag, and test the thickness of the ice cream with a spoon. Continue shaking for another few minutes until the desired thickness is achieved and enjoy! To really firm it up, place the ice cream in the freezer for a further 20 minutes.

⟨ ⟩ Olivia's Green Tea Blast Cupcakes ⟨ ⟩

My niece Olivia is 10. She came up with this quick and easy green tea cupcake recipe that can be decorated with nearly any topping of your choice, including green tea ice cream, cream cheese with almonds or pistachios, or a simple raspberry.

Ingredients

2 ½ cups of all-purpose flour

2 ½ tsp of baking powder

8 tbsp/4 oz of unsalted butter (room temperature)

1 ¼ cups of sugar

2 large eggs

2 ¼ tsp vanilla essence

1 ¼ cups of whipping cream

2 ½ tbsp of sweetened green tea powder

16 blackberries or raspberries.

Makes 16 servings.

Directions

1. Preheat oven to 350° F.
2. Place paper cases into two muffin pans.
3. Sift flour and baking powder in a bowl.
4. In a separate bowl, cream the butter, sugar, and then gradually add the eggs.
5. Pour the cream into a separate bowl and add the vanilla essence.
6. Add ⅓ of the flour mixture into the butter and egg mix.
7. Add ⅓ of the cream to the butter and egg mix. Continue to add the flour mix and cream to the butter and egg until blended. Whisk until smooth. *Continued on next page*

8. When smooth, finish by adding the green tea, and whisk to blend.

9. Scoop 1 tablespoon of the batter into each paper case until two thirds full.

10. Bake for 20-25 minutes until lightly golden, and the sponge bounces back when touched. A skewer inserted in the center should come out clean. You will see the lovely bright green color of tea showing through.

11. Transfer to a cake rack to cool slightly. These cupcakes are best eaten warm with a scoop of green tea ice cream!

Green Tea Truffles

Delicious served with a brandy refresher cocktail for parties, or have the children make their own chocolate balls for a fun and somewhat healthy treat to eat with a delicious frozen matcha.

Ingredients
½ lb of quality baking milk chocolate
3 tsp of *matcha* green tea powder
1 tbsp of full fat milk
¼ cup heavy cream
Matcha powder for coating

Directions:
1. Put 2 tsp of *matcha* powder in a small bowl; pour in warmed milk *matcha* and stir. Set to one side.
2. Finely chop chocolate in a medium bowl and warm in microwave for 2 minutes. Don't stir the chocolate; just watch it melt. You may only need to keep it in there for a minute, so keep an eye on it and don't let it burn.
3. Pour heavy cream into a small pan and heat gently on medium. Before it boils, stir in the *matcha* liquid thoroughly.
4. Pour the liquid over the chocolate, stirring gently.
5. Cool the chocolate at room temperature until it hardens, and then store it in the refrigerator for a final 10 minutes. This makes the chocolate easier to manage.
6. Scoop the chocolate into small 1 inch balls, working quickly to mold them with your hands, and place them on a sheet covered in foil. Cool in the refrigerator again for about 1 hr.
7. Once firm, turn and round the chocolate balls again, and dip them into green tea powder, coating evenly.

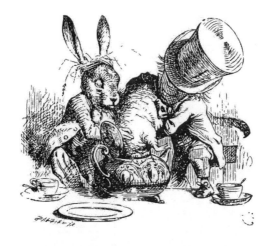

"Take some more tea," the March Hare said to
Alice, very earnestly.
"I've had nothing yet," Alice replied in an
offended tone, "so I can't take more."
"You mean you can't take *less*," said the Hatter:
"it's very easy to take *more* than nothing..."

Lewis Carroll, Alice in Wonderland

Suppliers

Naturopathic Doctors:

UK – Dr. Roderick Lane N.D.
Web: www.rodericklane.co.uk
Tel: London Clinic: 0845 0943224

US – Jacqueline Kidd Ph.D., N.P.
Director, Calabasas Center for Natural Health.
Web: www.calabasascenter.com
Tel: (818) 222 0422

Glass and Plastic Bottles, Pumps and Sprays Supplies

Nicola has used each of these suppliers over the years with great success:

ED Luce Packaging
Tel: (562) 802 0515
Web: www. Essentialsupplies.com

Sunburst Bottle
Tel: (877) 925 4500
Web: www.sunburstbottle.com

SKS Bottle and Packaging
Tel: (518) 880 6980
Web: www.sks-bottle.com

For high quality protective violet glass bottles, contact:

Miron Glass USA – Los Angeles, California
Tel: (323) 467 0558
Web: www. miron-glas.com/en/America

Essential Oil Suppliers:

Therapeutic grade essential oils best suited for teas and skincare:

Aroma Therapeutix
Tel: (1-800) 308 6284
Web: www.aromatherapeutix.com

Amrita Aromatherapy
Tel: (1-800) 410 9651
Web: www.amrita.net

doTerra Essential Oils
www.mydoterra.com/aroma1

Tisserand Aromatherapy
UK: 011441 273 325666
www.tisserand.com
www.tisserandusa.com

Essential oils for fragrancing rooms, body mists, room mists and sweet almond oil:

Liberty Natural Products
Tel: (1-800) 289 8427
Web: www.libertynatural.com

Dried Herbs and Loose Herbal Tea Suppliers:

Monterey Bay Spice Co
Tel: (831) 722 3400
Web: www. herbco.com

Mountain Rose Herbs
Tel: (1-800) 879 3337
Web: www.mountainroseherbs.com

Rosewater and Orange Blossom Water Suppliers:

Ethnicgrocer.com
Kalamala.com
Shamra.com

Pure Hibiscus Tea Suppliers:

Amazon.com
Flordejamaicasupplier.com
Nilevalleyherbs.com

Selected Tea Suppliers:

Adagioteas.com
Alvita.com
Arborteas.com
Bigelowtea.com
Bonavita.com
Celestialseasonings.com
Coffeebean.com
Compassiontea.com
Cost Plus/World Market.com

Harney.com

Jacksonsofpiccadilly.co.uk

Japanesegreenteaonline.com

Jenierteas.com

Living-qi.com

Matchasource.com

Mightyleaf.com

Numitea.com

Oolong-tea.org

Persimmontreetea.com

Revolutiontea.com

Rishi-tea.com

Smithtea.com

Starbucks.com

Taylorsofharrogate.com

Tazo.com

Teaforte.com

Teavana.com

Teaville.com

Teavivre.com

The Republic of Tea.com

TheTeaSpot.com

Traditionalmedicinals.com

Tripleleaf-tea.com

Tregothnan.co.uk

Twiningsusa.com

Whittard.com

World Flavorz.com

Yogiproducts.com

Yuuki-Cha.com

Zhitea.com

Tea Rooms

Los Angeles
Hotelbelair.com
Highteacottage.com
Thebeverlyhillshotel.com
Long Beach
Queenmary.com
San Diego
Thegranddelmar.com
Santa Barbara
Four Seasons Resort the Biltmore

For Tea Room Listings in the U.S.

Greattearoomsofamerica.com
Teamuse.com

For Tea Room Listings in the U.K.

Bettys.co.uk
Fortnumandmason.com
Theritzlondon.com
Fairmont.com

For an incredible number of delightful tea establishments you will find across the U.K. visit:
Findatearoom.co.uk

For lunches and afternoon teas in the U.K. at historical castles, abbeys, estates and homes visit:
www.nationaltrust.org.uk

Index

67, 69, 82, 84, 91, 92, 93, 102,
103, 109, 128, 129, 131, 132,
135, 138, 142, 144, 145, 146,
150, 156, 157, 161, 162, 166,
167, 179, 191, 194, 196, 197,
202, 205, 209, 211, 212, 215,
216, 217, 218, 221, 231, 238,
246, 258, 279
Body mist 157, 231, 258
Bones 59, 68, 166
Brandy refresher 240, 254
Breast cancer 68, 274, 275, 277, 281
Brewing 42, 46, 47, 62, 76, 78, 87,
93, 98, 123, 205
Bronchial congestion 103
Brucellosis bacteria 130
Buddhism 4, 12, 13, 14
Bulgarian rose 110, 183, 187, 189,
191
Butter tea 11, 19, 20, 22

C

Caffeine xiii, 25, 28, 37, 38, 44, 45,
46, 47, 48, 51, 55, 57, 61, 64,
67, 70, 72, 78, 81, 108, 179,
182, 195, 196, 200, 211, 212,
213, 225, 227, 277, 281
Calcium 53, 55, 59, 92, 106, 107
Calm 62, 86, 89, 99, 102, 111, 119,
131, 135, 136, 140, 143, 150,
156, 164, 183, 199, 211, 232
Camellia sinensis 9, 37, 38, 278, 279
Cancer 53, 54, 59, 61, 66, 67, 68, 69,
72, 91, 93, 94, 105, 109, 130,
131, 196, 197, 274, 275, 276,
277, 278, 279, 280, 281, 282,
284
Candida 142, 197
Candle diffuser 141, 156

Cardamom 29, 166, 227, 230, 241
Case Western Reserve University
School of Medicine 106
Cellulite 139, 220, 221, 222
Cellulitis 139
Ceylon 8, 52, 53
Chai 4, 11, 28, 29, 31, 53, 166, 167,
225, 241, 245
Chai Kahlua 241
Chakras 162, 167
Chamomile roman 135, 136, 165,
171, 175, 199, 232
Child birth 107
Chills 116
Chocolate Chai 245
Cholesterol 56, 67, 70, 71, 94, 97,
104, 105, 197, 275, 283
Chypre 175
Cinnamon 29, 97, 109, 132, 146,
166, 197, 233, 241, 245
Citrus 123, 128, 135, 138, 139, 146,
171, 172, 173, 175, 231, 234,
235
Clear spray 234
Clove 29, 94, 116, 123, 131, 137,
141, 146, 166, 206, 233
CO2 extraction 129
Cocktails vii, 237
Cold pressed 128
Colds and flu 115
Cold sores 100, 101, 142, 184
Colic 96, 103
Colitis 103
Comfort eating 139
Constipation 104, 225
Coronary Heart Disease 54, 59
Coughs 102, 103
Cranberry Fruit 90
Cranberry Gin Marteani 239
Crohn's disease 93

D

Dalai Lama 19
Dandelion 89, 91, 92
Darjeeling 33, 52
Decaffeinated 45, 47, 48, 51
Decoctions 87
Detox baths 221
Diabetes 59, 68, 93, 109, 273
Diabetes Type 1 93
Diabetes Type 2 59, 68, 109, 273
Diarrhea 55, 67, 104, 107, 226
Diastolic pressure 98
Digestion 25, 30, 55, 56, 82, 89, 92, 111, 135, 136, 224, 225, 283
Disruption 38
Diverticulitis 103
Dizziness 54, 67, 93, 96, 212
DNA 53, 71, 105, 283
Doctor Hsueh-Kung Lin 130
Dried florets 100
Dried herbs 81, 84, 101, 104, 127, 259
Drying herbs 86

E

Earl Grey 52, 123
Echinacea 89, 92, 93, 205, 206
Eczema 59, 109, 184
EGCGs 64
Egyptian 96, 103, 285
Eisai 4, 15, 16
Electric diffuser 156
Emotions 132, 149, 171, 234
English Breakfast 52, 53
Ernst J. Schaefer 54
Essential oil blends for teas 145

Essential oils xiii, xiv, xvii, xviii, xxi, xxii, 39, 53, 83, 120, 121, 124, 126, 127, 128, 129, 130, 131, 132, 133, 140, 144, 145, 146, 147, 150, 151, 152, 154, 155, 157, 161, 162, 163, 164, 165, 166, 167, 170, 171, 172, 173, 174, 175, 176, 179, 183, 185, 186, 187, 188, 201, 202, 205, 206, 207, 209, 211, 212, 213, 215, 217, 218, 219, 221, 225, 226, 228, 231, 232, 233, 234, 235, 258, 285
Eucalyptus 131, 137, 141, 142, 205, 206
Euphoric oils 153
Excessive acidity 59
Eyesight 56

F

Facemask 189
Fatigue 29, 100, 154, 212
Fennel 29, 132, 218
Fermentation 39, 55
Fever 95, 131
Fixation 39
Flavonoids 37, 53, 89, 195
Floral xvii, 34, 52, 110, 124, 173, 174, 175, 234
Flor de Jamaica 97
Flowers xix, xxii, 34, 39, 52, 71, 87, 89, 90, 97, 99, 100, 101, 126, 128, 132, 134, 136, 145, 169, 175, 179, 180, 200, 211, 213, 232, 234, 247
Flower Tea 34, 235
Flu 82, 93, 95, 101, 106, 115, 116, 130, 137, 142, 205, 206

Selected Bibliography

Authors & Sources:
- *Herbs Demystified*, Holly Phaneuf PhD.
- *The Encyclopedia of Medicinal Plants,* Andrew Chevalier
- www.plant-medicine.com
- Tea Association of the USA - www.teausa.com
- UK Tea Council - www.tea.co.uk
- International Tea Committee - www.intea.com

Black Tea and Pu'erh References:

Pub Med: *A thought on the biological activities of black tea. Plantation Products, Spices and Flavour,*
Technology Department, Central Food Technological Research Institute, Mysore, India.

Medline Plus
www.nim.nih.gov/medlineplus.com

Comparative studies on the hypolipidemic and growth suppressive effects of oolong, black, pu-erh, and green tea leaves in rat,.
Kuo KL, Weng MS, Chiang CT, Tsai YJ, Lin-Shiau SY, Lin JK.
Journal of agricultural and food chemistry, 2005 Jan 26;53(2):480-9.) Pub Med.

Pu-erh Tea Definition:
(http://en.wikipedia.org/wiki/Pu-erh_tea)

Chinese Natural Cures: Traditional Methods for Remedies and Preventions
Henry C. Lu.
Tess Press, 1994:14-15
Free radical scavenging effect of Pu-erh tea extracts and their protective effect on oxidative damage in human fibroblast cells,
Jie G, Lin Z, Zhang L, Lv H, He P, Zhao B.
Journal of agricultural and food chemistry, 2006 Oct 18;54(21):8058-

Oolong Tea References:

Pub Med: *Antihyperglycemic effect of oolong tea in Type 2 diabetes.*
Hosoda K, Wang MF, Liao ML, Chuang CK, Iha M, Clevidence B, Yamamoto S.
Research Center, Suntory, Osaka, Japan. Abstract: OBJECTIVE: To determine the efficacy of Oolong tea for lowering plasma glucose in type 2 diabetic patients in Miaoli, Taiwan.

United States Department of Agriculture
Agriculture Research Service. www.ars.usda.gov

Green Tea References:

www.greenteabase.com
www.wellnessresources.com

McKay DL, Blumberg JB: *The role of tea in human health: An update.*
J Am Coll Nutr 2002, **21**:1-13. PubMed Abstract
Kavanagh KT, Hafer LJ, Kim DW, Mann KK, Sherr DH, Rogers AE, Sonenshein

Green tea extracts decrease carcinogen-induced mammary tumor burden in rats and rate of breast cancer cell proliferation in culture.
J Cell Biochem 2001, **82**:387–398. PubMed Abstract | Publisher Full Text
Sueoka N, Suganuma M, Sueoka E, Okabe S, Matsuyama S, Imai K, Nakachi K, Fujiki H

A new function of green tea: prevention of lifestyle-related diseases.
Ann N Y Acad Sci 2001, **928**:274–280. PubMed Abstract | Publisher Full Text
Dona M, Dell'Aica I, Calabrese F, Benelli R, Morini M, Albini A, Garbisa

Neutrophil restraint by green tea: inhibition of inflammation, associated angiogenesis, and pulmonary fibrosis.
J Immunol 2003, **170**:4335–4341. PubMed Abstract | Publisher Full Text
Haqqi TM, Anthony DD, Gupta S, Ahmad N, Lee MS, Kumar GK, Mukhtar H:

Prevention of collagen-induced arthritis in mice by a polyphenolic fraction from green tea.
Proc Natl Acad Sci USA 1999, **96**:4524–4529. PubMed Abstract | Publisher Full Text | PubMed Central Full Text
Sudano Roccaro A, Blanco AR, Giuliano F, Rusciano D, Enea V:

Epigallocatechin-gallate enhances the activity of tetracycline in staphylococci by inhibiting its efflux from bacterial cells.
Antimicrob Agents Chemother 2004, **48**:1968–1973. PubMed Abstract | Publisher Full Text | PubMed Central Full Text
Sartippour MR, Shao ZM, Heber D, Beatty P, Zhang L, Liu C, Ellis L, Liu W, Go VL, Brooks MN

Green tea inhibits vascular endothelial growth factor (VEGF) induction in human breast cancer cells.
J Nutr 2002, **132**:2307-2311. PubMed Abstract | Publisher Full Text
Osada K, Takahashi M, Hoshina S, Nakamura M, Nakamura S, Sugano M

Tea catechins inhibit cholesterol oxidation accompanying oxidation of low density lipoprotein in vitro.
Comp Biochem Physiol Part C Toxicol Pharmacol 2001, **128**:153-164. Publisher Full Text
Weber JM, Ruzindana-Umunyana A, Imbeault L, Sircar

Inhibition of adenovirus infection and adenain by green tea catechins.
Antiviral Res 2003, **58**:167-173. PubMed Abstract | Publisher Full Text
Weinreb O, Mandel S, Amit T, Youdim MBH

Neurological mechanisms of green tea polyphenols in Alzheimer's and Parkinson's diseases.
J Nutr Biochem 2004, **15**:506-516. PubMed Abstract | Publisher Full Text
Raederstorff DG, Schlachter MF, Elste V, Weber P

Effect of EGCG on lipid absorption and plasma lipid levels in rats.
J Nutr Biochem 2003, **14**:326-332. PubMed Abstract | Publisher Full Text
Naghma K, Hasan M

Tea polyphenols for health promotion.
Life Sciences 2007, **81**:519-533. PubMed Abstract | Publisher Full Text
Moyers SB, Kumar NB

Green tea polyphenols and cancer chemoprevention: multiple mechanisms and endpoints for phase II trials.
Nutr Rev 2004, **62**:204-211. PubMed Abstract | Publisher Full Text
Mandel S, Weinreb O, Amit T, Youdim MB

Cell signaling pathways in the neuroprotective actions of the green tea polyphenol(-)-epigallocatechin-3-gallate: implications for neurodegenerative diseases.
J Neurochem 2004, **88**:1555-1569. PubMed Abstract | Publisher Full Text
Higdon JV, Frei B

Tea catechins and polyphenols: health effects, metabolism, and antioxidant functions.
Crit Rev Food Sci Nutr 2003, **43**:89-143. PubMed Abstract | Publisher Full Text
Xiang YZ, Shang HC, Gao XM, Zhang BL

Sato T, Miyata G: *The nutraceutical benefit, part I: green tea.*
Nutrition 2000, **16**:315-317. PubMed Abstract | Publisher Full Text
Belitz DH, Grosch W: *Qui'mica de los Alimentos.* Zaragoza: Acribia; 1997.
Graham HN

Green tea composition, consumption, and polyphenol chemistry.
Prev Med 1992, **21**:334-350. PubMed Abstract | Publisher Full Text
Vinson JA:

Beneficial Effects of Green tea: A literature Review by Sabu M Chacko, Priya, T Thambi, Ramadasan Kuttan and Ikuo Nishigaki shared interesting findings of the articles they read and reached consensus after discussion on available scientific research, a total of 105 peer-reviewed papers.

Black and green tea and heart disease: a review.
Biofactors 2000, **13**:127-132. PubMed Abstract | Publisher Full Text
Sano M, Tabata M, Suzuki M, Degawa M, Miyase T, Maeda-Yamamoto M:

Simultaneous determination of twelve tea catechins by high-performance liquid chromatography with electrochemical detection.
Analyst 2001, **126**:816-820. PubMed Abstract | Publisher Full Text
Khokhar S, Magnusdottir SGM

Total phenol, catechin, and caffeine contents of teas commonly consumed in the United Kingdom.
J Agric Food Chem 2002, **50**:565-570. PubMed Abstract | Publisher Full Text
Fernandez PL, Martin MJ, Gonzalez AG, Pablos F

A Review of the Health Effects of Green tea Catechins in In Vivo Animal Models.
J Nutr 2004, **134**:3431S-3440S. PubMed Abstract | Publisher Full Text
Roomi MW, Ivanov V, Kalinovsky T, Niedzwiecki A, RathIn M:

In vitro and in vivo antitumorigenic activity of a mixture of lysine, proline, ascorbic acid, and green tea extract on human breast cancer lines MDA-MB-231 and MCF-7.
Medical Oncol 2007, **22**(2):129-138. Publisher Full Text
Babu PV, Sabitha KE, Shyamaladevi CS:

Therapeutic effect of green tea extract on oxidative stress in aorta and heart of streptozotocin diabetic rats.
Chem Biol Interact 2006, **162**:114-120. PubMed Abstract | Publisher Full Text
Unno K, Takabayashi F, Yoshida H, Choba D, Fukutomi R, Kikunaga N, Kishido T, Oku N, Hoshino M:

Pharmacological effects of green tea on the gastrointestinal system.
Eur J Pharmacol 2004, **500**:177-185. PubMed Abstract | Publisher Full Text
Zaveri NT:

Green tea and its polyphenolic catechins: medicinal uses in cancer and noncancer applications.
Life Sci 2006, **78**:2073-2080. PubMed Abstract | Publisher Full Text
Tsuneki H, Ishizuka M, Terasawa M, Wu JB, Sasaoka T, Kimura I:

Effect of green tea on blood glucose levels and serum proteomic patterns in diabetic (db/db) mice and on glucose metabolism in healthy humans.
BMC Pharmacol 2004, **4**:18-21. PubMed Abstract | BioMed Central Full Text | PubMed Central Full Text
Meydani M:

Nutrition interventions in aging and age associated disease.
Ann N Y Acad Sci 2001, **928**:226-235. PubMed Abstract | Publisher Full Text
Mukhtar H, Wang ZY, Katlya SK, Agarwal R:

Tea components: antimutagenic and anticarcinogenic effects.
Prev Med 1992, **21**:351-360. PubMed Abstract | Publisher Full Text
Sano M, Takahashi Y, Yoshino K, Shimoi K, Nakamura Y, Tomita I, Oguni I, Konomoto H:

Effect of tea (Camellia sinensis L.) on lipid peroxidation in rat liver and kidney: a comparison of green and black tea feeding.
Biol Pharm Bull 1995, **18**:1006-1008. PubMed Abstract
Hara Y: **Advances in Food Science and Technology.** In *Nippon Shokuhin Kogyo.* Tokyo: Gakkai: Korin; 1990.
Shim JS, Kang MH, Kim YH, Roh JK, Roberts C, Lee IP:

Chemopreventive effect of green tea (Camellia sinensis) among cigarette smokers.
Cancer Epidemiol Biomarkers 1995, **4**:387-391.
McKay DL, Blumberg JB:

The role of tea in human health: an update.
J Am Coll Nutr 2002, **21**:1-13. PubMed Abstract | Publisher Full Text
Lu H, Meng X, Li C, Sang S, Patten C, Sheng S, Hong J, Bai N, Winnik B, Ho CT, Yang CS:

Glucuronides of tea catechins: enzymology of biosynthesis and biological activities.
Drug Metab Dispos 2003, **31**:452-461. PubMed Abstract | Publisher Full Text
Wu CH, Lu FH, Chang CS, Chang TC, Wang RH, Chang CJ:

Relationship among habitual tea consumption, percent body fat, and body fat distribution.
Obes Res 2003, **11**:1088-1095. PubMed Abstract | Publisher Full Text
Takabayashi F, Harada N, Yamada M, Murohisa B, Oguni I:

Inhibitory effect of green tea catechins in combination with sucralfate on Helicobacter pylori infection in Mongolian gerbils.
J Gastroenterol 2004, **39**:61-63. PubMed Abstract | Publisher Full Text
Yee YK, Koo MWL, Szeto ML:

Chinese tea consumption and lower risk of Helicobacter infection.
J Gastroenterol Hepatol 2002, **17**:552-555. PubMed Abstract | Publisher Full Text
Toda M, Okubo S, Ohnishi R, Shimamura T:

Antibacterial and bactericidal activities of Japanese green tea.
Nippon Saikingaku Zasshi 1989, **44**:669-672. PubMed Abstract
Mukoyama A, Ushijima H, Nishimura S, Koike H, Toda M, Hara
Y, Shimamura T:

Inhibition of rotavirus and enterovirus infections by tea extracts.
Jpn J Med Sci Biol 1991, **44**:181-186. PubMed Abstract
Yama TS, Shaha S, Hamilton-Millera JMT
Hirasawa M, Takada K:
Muraki S, Yamamoto S, Ishibashi H, Horiuchi T, Hosoi T, Suzuki
T, Orimo H, Nakamura K:
Effects of green tea extracts and polyphenols on the proliferation and activity of bone cells.
J Bone Miner Res 2003, **18**:S342.
Dorchies OM, Wagner S, Waldhauser KM, Buetler TM, Ruegg
UT

Potential therapeutic properties of green tea polyphenols in Parkinson's disease.
Drugs Aging 2003, **20**:711-721. PubMed Abstract | Publisher Full
Text
Sagesaka-Mitane Y, Miwa M, Okada S:

Platelet aggregation inhibitors in middle aged Japanese men and women.
Ann Epidemiol 1998, **7**:280-284.
Dvorakova K, Dorr RT, Valcic S, Timmermann B, Alberts DS:

Pharmacokinetics of the green tea derivative, EGCG, by the topical route of administration in mouse and human skin.
Cancer Chemother Pharmacol 1999, **43**:331-335. PubMed Abstract |
Publisher Full Text
Ishizuk H, Eguchi H, Oda T, Ogawa S, Nakagawa K, Honjo S,
Kono S:

Relation of coffee, green tea, and caffeine intake to gallstone disease in middle-age Japanese men.
Eur J Epidemiol 2003, **18**:401-405. PubMed Abstract | Publisher Full Text
Gupta SK, Halder N, Srivastava S, Trivedi D, Joshi S, Varma SD:

Green tea as a potent antioxidant in alcohol intoxication.
Addict Biol 2002, **7**:307-314. PubMed Abstract | Publisher Full Text
Ferrari CKB, Torres EAFS:

Biochemical pharmacology of functional foods and prevention of chronic diseases of aging.
Biomed Pharmacother 2003, **57**:251-260. PubMed Abstract | Publisher Full TextArburjai T, Natsheh FM:

Plants used in cosmetics.
Phytother Res 2003, **17**:987-1000. PubMed Abstract | Publisher Full Text
Min Zhang C, D'Arcy JH, Jiang-ping H, Xing X:

Green tea and the prevention of breast cancer: a case-control study in Southeast China.
Carcinogenesis 2005, **28**(5):1074-1078. Publisher Full Text
Zhang M, Holman CDAJ, Huang JP, Xie X

Impact of tea drinking on iron status in the UK: a review.
J Hum Nutr Diet 2004, **17**:43-54. PubMed Abstract | Publisher Full Text
Deng Z, Tao B, Li X, He J, Chen Y:

Health Benefits of White Tea References:

- American Chemical Society (14 August 2009). *"White Tea Could Keep You Healthy and Looking Young."* Science Daily. Retrieved 7 November 2010.
- American Chemical Society (13 April 2000). *"Cancer-Preventive Potential Of White Tea."* Science Daily. Retrieved 7 November 2010.
- Pace University (Fall 2004). *"Anti-viral, Anti-fungal and Anti-bacterial Effects of White Tea."*

Hibiscus References:

- Purdue University Horticulture & Landscape Architecture: Roselle Hibiscus sabdariffa L.; Morton, J.; 1987
- Journal of Nutrition: Hibiscus sabdariffa L. tea (tisane) lowers blood pressure in prehypertensive and mildly hypertensive adults; McKay DL; 2009
- Food and Chemical Toxicology: Hibiscus anthocyanins-rich extract inhibited LDL oxidation and oxLDL-mediated macrophages apoptosis; Chang YC; 2006
- Journal of Rheumatology: Treatment of fibromyalgia syndrome with Super Malic: a randomized, double blind, placebo controlled, crossover pilot study; Russell IJ; 1995
- Hibiscus.org: HIBISCUS: To Eat or Not to Eat?; Colleen Keena
- Bioscience, Biotechnology, and Biochemistry: Hibiscus Acid as an Inhibitor of Starch Digestion in the Caco-2 Cell Model System; Chanida HANSAWASDI; 2001

Lemon Balm References:

- Univeristy of Maryland Medical Center: American Ginseng "Neuropsychopharmacology."; Modulation of mood and cognitive performance following acute administration of single doses of Melissa officinalis (Lemon balm) with human CNS nicotinic and muscarinic receptor-binding properties; DO Kennedy et al; Octorber; 2003
  University of Maryland Medical Center :Lemon Balm
  Univeristy of Maryland Medical Center: Alzheimer's Disease

Pomegranate References:

- Mayo Clinic: Can Drinking Pomegranate Juice Help Lower My Cholesterol?
- Science Direct: Pomegranate Extract Improves a Depressive State
- Pomegranate Information: Discover the Power of Pomegranates
- ACAI Health and Nutrition Resource Center: Clinical evidence that pomegranates may slow Arthritis.
- Probelte Bio Laboratory in Spain for slowing down oxidation of DNA.

Raspberry Leaf References:

- J. Crow's; The Remarkable Raspberry, A good source of ellagic acid; Norma Whitehead
- Herbal Allies for Pregnancy Problems; Susun Weed
- American Pregnancy Association; Drinking herbal teas during pregnancy
- Getting Pregnant; Red Raspberry Leaf Tea – Fertility Tonic

Essential Oil References:

- www.roberttisserand.com
- Tea tree oil as an alternative topical decolonization agent for methicillin-resistant Staphylococcus aureus
  M. Caelli★, J. Porteous★, C. F. Carson†, R. Heller★ and T.V. Riley†
  ★Department of Clinical Epidemiology, University of Newcastle, Callaghan, NSW 2308 and
  †Department of Microbiology,The University of Western Australia, Nedlands,WA 6009, Australia
- MB Frank, Q Yang, HK Lin, et al., "Frankincense oil derived from Boswellia carteri induces tumor cell specific toxicity," BMC Complement Altern Med. 2009 Mar 18;9:6.
- T. Akihista, et al., "Cancer chemopreventive effects and cytotoxic activities of the triterpene acids from the resin of Boswellia carteri," Biol Pharm Bull. 2006 Sep;29(9):1976–9.
- M. Chevrier, et al., "Boswellia carteri Extract Inhibits TH1 Cytokines and Promotes TH2 Cytokines in Vitro," Clin Diagn Lab Immunol. 2005 May ;12(5):575–89.
- Juliet Highet, "Frankincense: Oman's Gift to the World." Prestel Publishing, 2006. 66.
- EJ Blain, et al., "Boswellia frereana (Frankincense) Suppresses Cytokine-Induced Matrix Metalloproteinase Expression and Production of Pro- Inflammatory Molecules in Articular Cartilage," Phytotherapy Research, 4:905-912 (2010).
- A. Frank, M. Unger, "Analysis of frankincense from various Boswellia species with inhibitory activity on human drug metabolizing cytochrome P450 enzymes using liquid chromatography mass spectrometry after utomated

on-line extraction," Journal of Chromatography A. 1112 (2006) 255–262.

- F. Nigel Hepper, "Arabian and African Frankincense Trees," Journal of Egyptian Archaeology. Vol. 55, (Aug., 1969), pp. 66–72.
- M. Thulin, A.M. Warfa, "The frankincense trees (Boswellia spp., Burseraceae) of northern Somalia and southern Arabia," Kew Bulletin. Vol. 42, No. 3 (1987), pp. 487–500.
- A. Moussaieff, et al., "Incensole acetate, an incense component, elicits psychoactivity by activating TRPV3 channels in the brain," The FASB Journal. 2008 Aug;22(8):3024–34.
- Antimicrobial activity of essential oils against Helicobacter pylori. Source Third Department of Internal Medicine, Kyoto Prefectural University of Medicine, Kyoto, 602-8566, Japan.
- Successful topical treatment of hand warts in a paediatric patient with tea tree oil (Melaleuca alternifolia). Millar BC, Moore JE. Source Northern Ireland Public Health Laboratory, Department of Bacteriology, Belfast, Ireland.
- Essential oil inhalation on blood pressure and salivary cortisol levels in prehypertensive and hypertensive subjects. Kim IH, Kim C, Seong K, Hur MH, Lim HM, Lee MS. Source College of Nursing, Eulji University, Daejeon, Republic of Korea.
- In Vitro Antibacterial Activity of Essential Oils against Streptococcus pyogenes.Sfeir J, Lefrançois C, Baudoux D, Derbré S, Licznar P.Source PRES LUNAM, Université d'Angers, Laboratoire de Bactériologie-Virologie, UFR Sciences Pharmaceutiques et Ingénierie de la Santé, 16 boulevard Daviers, 49045 Angers, Cedex 01, France.

The Power of Smell References:

- Sense of Smell Institute, Ltd. (1992). Living well with your sense of smell. New York, NY.
- Saeki Y and Mayumi S., Physiological effects of inhaling fragrances. The International Journal of Aromatherapy (2001), 11.3, 118-125.
- Haze S, Sakai K, and Gozu Y. Effects of fragrance inhalation on sympathetic activity in normal adults. Jpn. J. Pharmacol.(2002) 90, 247-253.
- Hongratanaworakit T and Buchbauer, G. Autonomic and emotional responses after transdermal absorption of sweet orange oil in humans: placebo controlled trial. International Journal of Essential Oil Therapeutics (2007) 1,29-34.
- Harris, B. Research reports: Harmonizing Ylang ylang. The International Journal of Aromatherapy (2005) 15, 54-57.
- Harris, B. Research reports: Menopausal treatment?. The International Journal of Aromatherapy (2006) 16.2, 101-104.
- Chen, SW.,Min L, Li WJ, Kong WX, Li JF, and Zhang YJ. The effects of angelica essential oil in three murine tests of anxiety. Pharmcol Biochem Behav. 2004 Oct;79(2):377-82.
- Ceccarelli I, Lariviere WR, Fiorenzani P, Aloisi AM. Effects of long-term exposure of lemon essential oil odor on behavioral, hormonal and neuronal parameters in male and female rates. Brain Res. 2004 Mar 19;1001(1-2):78-86.
- Park MK, Lee ES. The effect of aroma inhalation method on stress responses of nursing students. Dept. of Nursing, Nambu University, Gwangsan-gu, Gwangju city, Korea.

- Harris, B. Aromatherapy and Palliative Care: excerpts from the Essential Oil Research Database. The International Journal of Clinical Aromatherapy (2004) Vol 1, Issue 2, 51-53.
- Hansen, TM. Hansen B. and Ringdal GI. Does aromatherapy massage reduce job-related stress? Results from a randomized, controlled trial. The International Journal of Aromatherapy (2006) 16,89-94.

Picture Credits

Royalty Free Photography - 123RF.com

Olena Ovcharenko – Geisha and Sakura., Kenneth Valles - Organic tea leaves after a rainstorm; Sezefei – Tea plantations at Cameron Highlands Malaysia.; Omela – Cup of Tea; Lian2011 – Tea Ceremony in Japanese Style; Braden Gunem – Hands of a Tibetan monk holding a wooden tea cup, Lama Yuru, Ladakh India; Irina Belousa – Traditional Moroccan Mint Tea; Alexander Romanov – Russian Samovar Painted in Folk Style; Birute Vijeikiene – Still Life with Different Spice and Brassy Quern; Valentyn Volkov – Cloves, Anise and Cinnamon; Ruth Black – Afternoon Tea; Leonid Shcheglov – Three Tea Flowers; Serezniy – Exotic Green Tea wit Flowers in Glass Teapot; Worradirek Muksab – Tea Plantation on Hill with Worker Harvest; Birute Vijeikiene – Tea Assortment Around the White Cup of Tea; Hamsterman – Green Leaf Tea versus Coffee Beans in Yin Yang Shaped Plate; Marcin Chodorowski – Drop of Tea; Annete – Black Loose Tea; Glock33 – Oolong Green Chinese Tea; Ingridhs – Tea Collection – Bancha and Sencha Green Tea and Matcha Green Tea; 91010ra – Powdered Green Tea; Alex Burmakin – Japanese Geisha; Maksim Shebeko – Traditional Tea Ceremony Accessories (Japan); Martina Osmy – Herbs for Medicine; George Tsartisiandidis – Fresh Herbs Hanging on a Rope; Olga Miltsova – Mortar with Herbs Isolated; Natalia Khlapsuhyna – Healing Herbs in Glass Bottles; Vesna Cvorovic – Chamomile Tea; Monica Adamczyk – Cup of Cranberry Tea; Ingridhs – Dandelion Tea; Lilyana Vynogradova – Echinacea Purpurea Flower; Belchonock – Young Garlic; Anton Agnatenco – Hot Ginger Tea with Lemon and

Honey; Yuri Minaev – Hibiscus – Flower, Dry Tea and Brewed Tea in a Teapot; Firina – Two Cups of Lavender Tea and a Bunch of Fresh Lavender; Martina Osmy – Lemon Balm Leaves with Pestle and Mortar; Marco Mayer – Iced Tea; Natika – Ripe Pomegranate Piece; Sereziny - Ripe Raspberries with Mint; Oksana Bratanova – Rooibos Tea; Monica Adamczyk – Dried Roses; Marco Mayer – Spiced Tea; Nito500 – Lavender Flowers; Ivan Kmit – Drop from Leaf to Bottle; Dmitry Kovalenko – Aromatherapy Oil and Rose Flower; George Tsartsiandidis – Herbs and Spices on a Wooden Palette; Marilyn Barbone – Herb Leaf Selection; Roman Malanchuk – Rose Belchonock – Bottles with Ingredients; Ying Feng Johansson – Close up of Lotus Flower; Jhetta – Bottles of Essential Oils; Andreja Donko – Dry Lavender on an Old Book; Natalia Klenova – Cup of Green Tea and White Towel; George Tsartsiandidis – Cup of Verbena; Olga Miltsova – Honey and Tea; Juergen Priewe – The Beauty of Hibiscus; Sandra Cunningham – Enjoying a Good Cup of Tea in the Morning; Piccia Neri – Beautiful Chamomile Flowers Picked Up in a Field; Robyn Mackenzie – Bag of Dried Lavender; Dmitry Lobanov – Martini Alcohol Cocktails; Madllen – Ice Cream

CPSIA information can be obtained
at www.ICGtesting.com
Printed in the USA
FFOW03n1942280114
3318FF